TREATING ACNE

TREATING ACNE

RICHARD A. WALZER, M.D.
and the Editors of Consumer Reports Books

CONSUMER REPORTS BOOKS
A DIVISION OF CONSUMERS UNION
Yonkers, New York

Copyright © 1992 by Richard A. Walzer

Published by Consumers Union of United States, Inc., Yonkers, New York 10703.

All rights reserved, including the right of reproduction in whole or in part in any form.

LIBRARY OF CONGRESS CATALOGING-IN-PUBLICATION DATA

Walzer, Richard A., 1930–
    Treating acne : a guide for teens and adults / Richard A. Walzer
and the editors of Consumer Reports Books.
      p. cm.
    Includes index.
    ISBN 0-89043-449-2
    1. Acne—Popular works.   I. Consumer Reports Books.   II. Title.
RL131.W35   1992
616.5′3—dc20   91-40262
                                                      CIP

Design by Kathryn Parise
Drawings by Vaune J. Hatch
First printing, February 1992

Manufactured in the United States of America

Treating Acne is a Consumer Reports Book published by Consumers Union, the nonprofit organization that publishes *Consumer Reports*, the monthly magazine of test reports, product Ratings, and buying guidance. Established in 1936, Consumers Union is chartered under the Not-for-Profit Corporation Law of the State of New York.

The purposes of Consumers Union, as stated in its charter, are to provide consumers with information and counsel on consumer goods and services, to give information on all matters relating to the expenditure of the family income, and to initiate and to cooperate with individual and group efforts seeking to create and maintain decent living standards.

Consumers Union derives its income solely from the sale of *Consumer Reports* and other publications. In addition, expenses of occasional public service efforts may be met, in part, by nonrestrictive, noncommercial contributions, grants, and fees. Consumers Union accepts no advertising or product samples and is not beholden in any way to any commercial interest. Its Ratings and reports are solely for the use of the readers of its publications. Neither the Ratings, nor the reports, nor any Consumers Union publications, including this book, may be used in advertising or for any commercial purpose. Consumers Union will take all steps open to it to prevent such uses of its material, its name, or the name of *Consumer Reports*.

Contents

	Introduction	1
1 ■	What Is Acne?	5
2 ■	Causes of Acne	17
3 ■	Treatment: Self-Help	27
4 ■	Treatment: Seeing a Dermatologist	39
5 ■	Cosmetics	59
6 ■	Repairing the Damage: Scars	67
7 ■	If It's Not Acne, What Is It?	81
8 ■	Finding Professional Help	89
	Glossary	93
	Index	95

The information contained in this book is not intended to substitute for professional or medical advice. Consumers Union disclaims responsibility or liability for any loss that may be incurred as a result of the use or application of any information included in *Treating Acne*. Readers should always consult their physicians or other professionals for treatment and advice. The editors have exercised meticulous care to ensure the accuracy and timeliness of the information in this book. The information contained herein concerning brand names and product formulations was based on the latest available as we went to press. Readers should keep in mind that product names and formulas may change from time to time, that the products mentioned in this book were not tested by Consumers Union, and that their inclusion in the text does not imply endorsement by Consumers Union.

TREATING
ACNE

Introduction

Acne is by no means a new human affliction. The origin of the word that describes eruptions on the faces of adolescents dates back more than two thousand years. In ancient Greece the word *acme*, meaning "point or peak," was applied to puberty, then considered to be the peak of life. The word *acne* evolved as a distortion of *acme*, and the facial blemishes that appeared at the time of acme were called "acnes."

Why write a book on this easily identifiable problem that we have experienced for thousands of years? There are three compelling reasons. First, acne is by far the most common skin disease and therefore one of the most common diseases affecting us. Eighty percent of any human population will experience some manifestation of acne. Twenty-five percent of them will have acne serious enough to merit some form of treatment, professional or otherwise.

Second, the social, economic, and psychological effects of acne can be painful. Americans spend millions of dollars a year on acne treatments. For many sufferers, acne causes depression and gets in the way of social and sexual relationships. Society in general is prejudiced against people with acne; they are less likely to be offered jobs, for example.

Finally, misconceptions about the cause and treatment of acne are widespread, and they persist even in the face of scientific information to the contrary. Patients with acne commonly tell their doctors that:

Acne is caused by dirt and poor hygiene. Frequent and vigorous washing is good treatment.

Acne flare-ups are caused by emotional stress. If one can live a stress-free life, the condition of the skin will certainly improve.

Sexual activity is good/bad for the skin and excessive/infrequent sex causes blemishes to develop.

Certain foods cause acne breakouts. Avoiding these foods is essential to clear skin.

All of these mistaken notions show quite clearly that today's youth—and many older people as well—still cling to outmoded ideas about the causes and treatment of acne.

These and other questionable concepts are addressed in this book. Chapter 1 defines acne and describes the various skin eruptions that appear in the course of the disease. Unusual variants, such as infantile acne, are also discussed. Chapter 2 provides details of our current understanding of the causes of acne as well as some of the factors that may or may not influence the course of the disease.

Treatment is discussed in the chapters that follow. Chapter 3 deals with self-help treatments, including over-the-counter, nonprescription medications, whereas Chapter 4 considers professional treatment and the types and safe uses of prescription medications. Chapter 5 discusses the role of cosmetics in promoting acne as well as the kinds of cosmetics that are useful for the individual with oily skin and/or acne. The problem of treating the marks and scars left on the skin by severe acne is addressed in Chapter 6. Chapter 7 covers some skin diseases that might be mistaken for acne. The final chapter deals with finding the right doctor. A glossary follows of some of the scientific terms used.

Although new drugs and treatments are being developed all the time, this book contains the latest information on effective acne treatments available today. The important news, then, is that no one should have to suffer the embarrassment and trauma caused by this psychologically debilitating condition. Over-the-counter medications and professional treatment, if necessary, can make all the difference.

1

What Is Acne?

Acne is a skin disorder affecting the hair follicles and sebaceous glands on the face, chest, and back. Hair follicles are the tubelike structures that produce and hold the hair; the sebaceous glands attached to the hair follicles make an oily substance called "sebum," which lubricates and protects the surface of the skin (see Figure 1.1). The sebaceous gland is attached to the hair follicle by a tubular structure called a duct, which carries the gland's oily secretion into the hair follicle and then to the surface through a structure called the "pilosebaceous duct" (Figure 1.2). It is in and around the pilosebaceous duct that acne occurs.

The blemishes that make up acne take several different forms. This is in contrast to other skin conditions in which there is only one type of eruption—the rash of chicken pox is made up exclusively of small blisters, for example. Knowing the variety of blemishes that occur in acne is important, since it will help you to understand the causes of acne and why some treatments are more helpful than others.

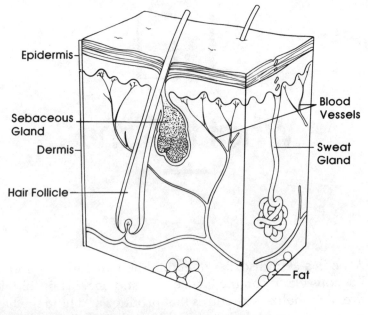

FIGURE 1.1 Cross section of the skin

TYPES OF ACNE SYMPTOMS
Comedones

The first blemish to form as acne begins to appear is called a "comedone," and it is critical to all the blemishes that eventually develop. A comedone is a plug that forms within the pilosebaceous duct. It is made up of dead cells from the lining of the duct that are mixed with sebum produced by the oil gland (Figure 1.3).

There are two types of comedones. The *open comedone*, more familiarly called a blackhead, is visible on the skin because the plug has formed in the surface opening of the duct (Figure 1.4). Blackheads are not black because of dirt; they take their color from the normal skin pigment that is within the dead cells. The other type of comedone, the *closed comedone* or whitehead, is a similar plug within the duct, but it is located deeper, underneath the skin's surface

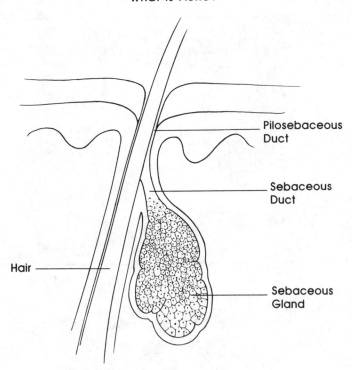

FIGURE 1.2 The sebaceous gland and duct

(Figure 1.5). Closed comedones appear as small, pale elevations, without any obvious openings.

Blackheads can usually be eliminated by gentle squeezing; whiteheads are difficult to remove, requiring a puncture to open them and considerable pressure to push out their contents. (The pros and cons of attempting to remove comedones is discussed in detail in later chapters.) Blackheads are unsightly, but it is the closed comedone that is responsible for other blemishes that may develop.

Papules

The word *papule* is synonymous with the word *pimple*. Papules are firm, red swellings of various sizes that appear

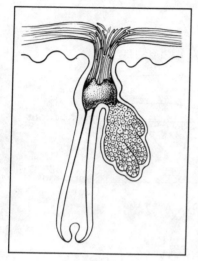

FIGURE 1.3

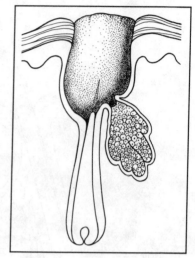

FIGURE 1.4

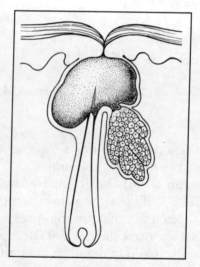

FIGURE 1.5

on normal skin as another manifestation of acne. Actually, most papules develop at the site of closed comedones, but the comedone may be so tiny that it can be seen only with a microscope. Sometimes papules are tender to the touch, but more often they are not. Squeezing will not eliminate

What Is Acne?

a papule because it is solid and there is nothing to squeeze out. In fact, vigorous squeezing may injure the skin, increase inflammation in the area, and actually enlarge the papule. The best "first aid" treatments for papules are warm compresses and drying creams or lotions (see Chapter 3).

Pustules

Pustules are small abscesses on the skin. They are soft pimples filled with pus, which is made up of white blood cells. Pustules can be on the surface of the skin or deep within it. Those that are superficial break easily, either by themselves or by the process of washing, and they disappear quickly, within three or four days. Deeper pustules, indicating a more severe form of acne, are not easily broken and should not be squeezed. Very large and deep pustules sometimes have to be incised and drained by a dermatologist in order to prevent scarring.

Acne Cysts

Acne cysts are large areas of inflammation deep within the skin. Sometimes they are formed by two or more adjacent blemishes coming together to form a single, red, tender swelling. They are often filled with a thick, creamy fluid made up of pus, dead cells, and sebum. Acne cysts are responsible for most of the scarring associated with severe acne and consequently require professional attention.

Macules

After acne blemishes subside, flat, reddened areas frequently remain on the skin. These *macules* represent the end stage of the inflammatory process. Unfortunately, they add to the cosmetic problem and may persist for a long time, sometimes for months.

Hyperpigmentation

An increase in the brown skin pigment called melanin sometimes remains after acne blemishes have healed, as it often does in other forms of inflammation, such as sunburn. Like red macules, such hyperpigmentation is not permanent, although it may be months before it fades away. Bleaching creams are available but are not reliable and are best reserved for the rare situation in which the hyperpigmentation fails to disappear spontaneously.

Scars

Scars are permanent alterations in the normal structure of the skin. Many people with cystic acne develop scars because of the destruction of connective tissue in the deeper layers of skin. More surprising is the fact that some people with relatively superficial acne blemishes also develop scars. Thus, scarring seems to be an individual response to inflammation and tissue damage. Furthermore, the type of scar that forms can vary from person to person. One of the most obvious kinds of scar is called a keloid. This is a large, pink, often oddly shaped mound of thick scar tissue that forms at the site of the injury and subsequent healing. Strangely, the amount of scar tissue in keloids is not always proportionate to the severity of the acne, and seemingly minor blemishes may lead to large keloids. Keloids most often occur on the chest and back and less frequently on the face, jaw, or forehead.

Another common scar that can follow acne inflammation is called an "ice pick" scar. As the name implies, this is a deep, pointlike depression, as if a sharp object had been driven into the skin. Other scars may appear where skin tissue has been lost; these form depressed areas, as if a portion of the skin had been scooped out.

You should not assume that everyone who experiences acne will have all these different blemishes. It is not uncommon to have mostly one type and a scattering of some of the others. You might have comedone acne, in which the outbreak is almost entirely made up of blackheads and closed comedones; pustular acne, in which all the blemishes are pus pimples; or cystic acne, in which deep cysts predominate. Which treatment is best depends on the nature of the predominant blemish as well as on the overall severity of the problem.

Although all the varieties of acne have features in common, several unusual and distinctive forms of acne can be separated from the common adolescent types. These conditions affect disparate age groups—the very young and the adult.

INFANTILE ACNE

It is not uncommon for the symptoms of acne to appear on the cheeks and chin of infants some six to twelve weeks after birth. Usually the outbreak is mild, distressing to the parents perhaps but not troubling baby one bit. Generally the outbreak is superficial, with small papules and pustules predominating. Although the cause of infantile acne is not known, it appears to occur during a brief stage of postnatal development when the infant's sebaceous glands are very actively producing sebum. There is speculation that hormones produced during the mother's pregnancy are responsible for the increased oil gland activity and the resulting acne. (See Chapter 2 for a discussion of the hormonal influences on the sebaceous glands.)

Infantile acne affects boys more often than girls, and studies suggest that a family history of acne is a predisposing factor. Most cases clear up in a matter of weeks without any treatment; it is the rare case that continues for months, when treatment becomes an option. In such a case, the parents should remember that the baby is neither suffering from nor aware of the "problem." Most treatment, then, is for the benefit of the parents.

12　　　　　　　　　TREATING ACNE

Does the presence of infantile acne indicate that significant outbreaks will inevitably appear in adolescence? Probably not.

ADULT ACNE

At the other end of the chronological spectrum, there appears to be a growing population of adults who continue to experience acne long after it should have subsided. Still others may develop acne for the first time in their late twenties or thirties. A number of theories exist to explain this phenomenon, including changes in the environment, dietary factors such as additives and pollutants, and the impact of stress found in contemporary society. To be fair, no statistical studies actually confirm an increase in adult acne. It is quite possible that a growing cosmetic sophistication and an awareness of the new, more effective forms of treatment have increased the number of adults who seek medical help. In other words, persistent or adult-onset acne may have always been around but in the past was largely ignored or self-treated.

Whatever the reasons for the increase, affected women seem to outnumber men by a considerable margin. Many women with adult-onset acne show a distinctive pattern of eruptions, with most of the blemishes appearing over the jawbones and neck. This is in contrast to adolescent acne, in which the outbreaks are concentrated on the cheeks, chin, and forehead.

Adult acne is treated much the same way as other forms of acne. Two areas of acne treatment and control, however, have greater significance for adult women: hormonal regulation and the use of cosmetics (see Chapters 4 and 5).

ACNE CONGLOBATA

Acne conglobata is an unusually severe type of acne in which round (conglobate) collections of pus form deep in

What Is Acne?

the skin. These abscesses often develop next to each other and then unite into larger areas that seem to burrow under the skin, forming what are called "sinus tracts." The result of acne conglobata is considerable tissue destruction and large, irregularly shaped scars, particularly of the keloid variety.

The cause of this form of acne is unknown. Scientists speculate that something has gone wrong with the individual's ability to regulate and modulate the inflammation. Furthermore, it is one of the most difficult kinds of acne to treat. Some of the most potent drugs—antibiotics in large doses, corticosteroids, or isotretinoin—are usually required to halt the disease (see Chapter 4).

A fortunately rare form of acne conglobata called acne fulminans is characterized by its sudden onset and the fact that it is not only a skin disease but a systemic illness as well. People with acne fulminans experience fever, swelling and pain in their joints, and a general feeling of malaise. This form of acne is also poorly understood and difficult to treat.

OCCUPATIONAL ACNE

The work environment can frequently initiate acne or aggravate an acne condition that is already present. Teenagers who work in fast-food restaurants, where the air is filled with fine particles of cooking oil, may experience an outbreak of acne. Office workers who spend hours on the telephone have been known to develop a one-sided acne traced to the constant pressure and friction of the phone against the skin. Athletes can experience friction acne from chin guards, shoulder pads, or other tight-fitting equipment or uniforms. Sweating under athletic garb can also contribute to the acne problem.

One of the most important forms of occupational acne is often seen in industrial workers who are exposed to chemical compounds containing forms of chlorine and bromine. Known as chloracne, this condition may be caused by chemicals that were used in the past to manufacture electrical equipment, wire insulation, and plastics and are still found in insecticides and weed killers. Fortunately, casual or occasional exposure to these chemicals is not likely to cause an outbreak of acne.

The first line of treatment for all forms of occupational acne is to eliminate or modify the factors that are causing the condition—and the sooner the better. Treatment is not likely to be very successful in the face of continued exposure.

MEDICATION ACNE

It is well known that a number of medications can cause all sorts of skin rashes, either from an allergic reaction or from the toxic effects of the drug on the skin. A common example is the outbreak of hives (urticaria), frequently seen as a manifestation of an allergy to penicillin. So it is not surprising that acnelike reactions can also occur from other medications.

Certain hormonal drugs that directly or indirectly affect the sebaceous glands are among the most frequent offenders. Athletes and bodybuilders who take testosteronelike synthetic hormones called anabolic steroids to build up their muscles may experience acne as a side effect. This is because anabolic steroids are in fact androgenic (related to male hormones) and stimulate the oil glands. The cortisonelike hormones can also cause acne either from internal administration or through direct application to the skin. This is an interesting paradox, since these same corticosteroids are sometimes used to treat some severe forms of acne.

Birth control pills can incite or suppress acne, depending upon the relative amounts of estrogen, the female hormone, and progesterone, which may have male hormonelike effects that tend to stimulate the oil glands.

What Is Acne?

Some of the other frequently prescribed medications that may aggravate or initiate an acne breakout are lithium, widely used to treat depression; phenytoin, an anticonvulsant used to treat epilepsy and other forms of seizure disorders; isoniazid, a medication used to treat tuberculosis; and medications that contain iodine or bromine.

As in occupational acne, the most effective way of treating medication acne is the elimination of the medication causing it. Unfortunately this is not always possible. The medication may be critical to the individual's health, and there may not be another drug available that will do much the same thing without the undesirable side effect. When this is the case, the acne can be treated conventionally, but the outcome is unlikely to be very satisfactory.

There are other acne conditions that are sometimes singled out as distinctive, but for the most part these are instances where a case of conventional acne is influenced, usually for the worse, by a particular environmental, chemical, or physical factor.

2

Causes of Acne

Life would be considerably less complicated if every problem we confronted had a single cause and a single solution.
In the field of medicine, both doctors and patients could
better cope with illness if there were one identifiable cause
for each ailment. Unfortunately this is not the case. Consider, for example, a common infection, the streptococcal
sore throat. The streptococcus bacteria have to find their
way into a person's pharynx for the sore throat to develop,
but there are many people walking around with streptococcus bacteria living and multiplying in their pharynxes
who show no symptoms of the infection. It is obvious, then,
that other factors in addition to the presence of the bacteria make it possible for the strep throat to develop. Possible
changes in the body's immune status, appropriate local
conditions in the throat, as well as some unknown factors
all contribute to making the infection happen.

Much the same can be said for acne. Not every teenager
with oily skin has acne. Not every adolescent whose
mother and father had acne in their youth develops acne.
A good deal is known about the *pathogenesis* of acne (that
is, the way the disease develops), but it is still not always
possible to answer the question "Why do I have acne and

18   TREATING ACNE

my brother, sister, and friend do not?" Acne has many causes; some are readily identifiable, others are not.

WHY ACNE MAY HAPPEN
Genetic Factors

Circumstantial evidence exists that acne is in part a genetic, or inherited, disease. In studies of identical twins—twins that develop from one fertilized egg—if one twin had acne, 97 percent of the other co-twins had acne as well. In the case of nonidentical twins—or twins that develop from separate fertilized eggs—the figure was 50 percent. In other family studies, 80 percent of acne sufferers had a brother or sister similarly afflicted, and in 60 percent one or both parents had experienced acne while growing up. There is an impression among dermatologists that the severest cases of acne occur in those youngsters both of whose parents had acne or where one parent had very severe acne.

What does all this mean? It simply suggests that some unknown trait or factor can be passed on from parent to child that, in the presence of other existing factors, promotes the development of acne.

Oily Skin

Most people think that acne and oily skin go together. Generally speaking, this is true. As a group, people with acne do have oilier skin than individuals who do not. Furthermore, if you do have acne, the severity of the condition seems roughly to parallel the amount of oil on the skin surface—that is, the oilier your skin the worse your acne. Nevertheless, oily skin is not the *cause* of acne, since there are many sufferers who have normal or even dry skin and many, many people who have oily skin without a trace of acne. To add to the confusion, the acne can disappear and the oily skin remain.

Hormones

Hormones are substances that are produced in the body by the endocrine glands and are carried by the blood to other parts of the body where they act as chemical messengers and regulate various bodily functions. For example, the thyroid gland, located in the neck under the Adam's apple, manufactures and secretes a hormone called thyroxin, which regulates the metabolism, affecting such diverse functions as hair growth and the rate of heartbeat.

Androgens (male hormones) are the only hormones that directly stimulate oil glands to enlarge and produce sebum. But both sexes produce androgens: males in the testes and adrenal glands, and females in the ovaries and adrenal glands. Of course, there is a difference in the normal amounts of androgens produced by each sex. Since acne is associated with enlarged oil glands and oily skin, it seems likely, then, that androgens are important factors in the development of the disease.

In contrast, estrogens (female hormones) to some extent block the effects of androgens on the oil glands, reducing the size of the glands and the amount of oil produced. Of these two "opposing" hormones, androgens seem to be dominant, since relatively small amounts of androgens can overwhelm the action of even large amounts of estrogens. It is important to understand that the majority of people who have acne, both male and female, do *not* have abnormal amounts of these hormones for their age and sex. It may be that the sebaceous glands of people who have acne react differently, perhaps excessively, to normal amounts of these hormones in the body.

Some abnormal conditions, such as cysts or tumors of the adrenal or sex glands, can cause larger than normal amounts of androgens to be produced. When this occurs

20   TREATING ACNE

in women, they may experience an increase in facial and
body hair, a disturbance in their menstrual cycle, and
acne. Obviously, acne occurring in this situation is merely
a symptom of a more serious problem requiring the specialized attention of a gynecologist or endocrinologist.

The fact that (1) androgens stimulate the oil glands and
encourage acne to happen and that (2) estrogens to some
extent block this action has important consequences when
it comes to the treatment of acne in women (see Chapter
4).

Another group of hormones directly affects the sebaceous glands and therefore can influence the course of
acne. These are the *corticosteroids*, cortisonelike hormones made by the adrenal glands. Corticosteroids are
prescribed widely for the treatment of conditions ranging
from skin rashes to arthritis. Unfortunately, they sometimes activate the sebaceous glands, encouraging the development of acne, although it takes relatively large doses
of corticosteroids, taken for a period of weeks, to cause so-
called steroid acne. Similarly, the strong corticosteroid
creams, ointments, and lotions used by dermatologists to
treat many different skin conditions also can cause acne or
aggravate it, if it is already present.

Blockage of Follicles

The earliest event in the development of acne is the formation of the comedone, an oily plug that blocks the follicle opening on the skin surface (blackhead) or forms an
obstruction in the follicle underneath the skin surface
(whitehead). Under normal circumstances, the inside of
the follicle is lined with cells that are similar to the cells of
the surface layer of the skin, the epidermis. These cells
grow, mature, die, flake off, and are carried to the surface
of the skin by the flow of sebum. People with acne have a
defect in the behavior of these follicle-lining cells, which
results in their not flaking off in a normal manner. These

Causes of Acne 21

cells are not carried to the surface; instead they block the inside of the follicle, trapping oil and bacteria and forming a comedone.

Why the follicle-lining cells behave in this way in some people and not in others is a mystery, but attempting to correct this defect with medication is a basic part of acne treatment.

Bacteria

Acne is not an "infection" in the true sense of the word, but bacteria inside of the acne-susceptible follicles do contribute to acne inflammation. These bacteria feed on sebum and break up this complex oily material into smaller molecules called fatty acids. The acne bacteria and the fatty acids attract white blood cells from the bloodstream and nearby skin into the follicle. The white blood cells release chemicals that make holes in the walls of the follicle and allow the contents of the follicle—the sebum, dead cells, and bacteria—to leak out into the adjacent skin, creating a local inflammation. When the area of inflammation is large enough, we see it as a papule, pustule, or acne cyst.

The bacteria that play a role in acne are not strangers to human skin. They are part of the group of living organisms that are considered normal residents of the skin and are found in everyone's follicles. Nevertheless, reducing their number through treatment can effectively improve if not eliminate the acne.

ACNE MYTHS AND TRUTHS

It is clear that acne cannot be avoided by a little "preventive maintenance." For this reason both doctors and patients often focus their attention on several larger issues in which there is some potential to influence the course of the skin problem. These factors include skin hygiene, climate, diet, and stress.

Skin Hygiene

It can be said unequivocally that acne has nothing to do with "dirty" skin. As we have already learned, blackheads are *not* dirt but are impactions or collections of dead skin cells and oil found inside the follicle opening. Certainly acne-prone skin is apt to be oilier than healthy skin, but the bacteria living on the skin surface are much the same in people with acne as in those without acne. Moreover, the bacteria that are involved in the acne process live deep inside the follicle and sebaceous gland. Washing the skin frequently or vigorously does little to reduce the number of these acne bacteria or diminish their activity in acne inflammation.

Cleaning the skin as a form of treatment remains popular, but vigorous cleansing can actually make the acne worse by damaging the already weakened follicles.

Climate

Acne has no respect for climate or weather. The disease is found in all regions of the world, hot or cold, wet or dry. Sunny climes produce as many acne sufferers as the more temperate areas.

The long-held impression that natural sunlight is good treatment for acne is open to question for two reasons. First, only 50 percent of acne patients improve with sun exposure and tanning. The remaining 50 percent experience no change or a worsening of the condition. Sun-induced flare-ups of acne may occur because the sun causes a thickening of the skin, which can contribute to the blockage of follicles. In fact, "sun acne" on the back and shoulders is common among lifeguards and other people who spend a lot of time at the beach. Second, with the dramatic increase in all forms of skin cancer, which is thought to be related to excessive sun exposure, dermatologists are reluctant to treat acne with artificial ultraviolet light or en-

Causes of Acne 23

courage sunbathing, even for those who do notice improvement of their acne during the summer months.

High humidity is another climatic factor that can promote acne. Presumably it is caused by overhydration of the skin, as in the case of an ordinary heat rash, when the skin gets saturated with water and the sweat pores and follicles are blocked. In fact, high humidity rather than the sun may be the cause of some acne flare-ups in the summer.

Diet

It is difficult to eliminate the widespread belief that certain foods can cause acne. It is only in the past twenty years that doctors themselves have come to realize that diet has little to do with the development of the disease. However, many people still cling to the dietary factors as a probable cause of their acne because of the erratic behavior of the disease and the lack of a better explanation for sudden outbreaks.

The belief that chocolate causes acne was discarded years ago. A careful study of chocolate eaters versus those who do not eat chocolate revealed no difference in the severity of acne. Although very low calorie, starvation diets can markedly decrease the amount of sebum produced by the oil glands, in the normal dietary range there is no apparent relationship between calories consumed and the severity of acne. Furthermore the kinds of foods eaten—whether carbohydrates, fat, or protein—play no role in the development of acne.

Another common misconception suggests that an oily skin, a possible promoter of acne, is directly related to the amount of oil consumed in the diet. Thus, oily foods such as pizza and french fried potatoes should be taboo for individuals who are acne-prone. The reality is that the oil glands produce sebum in quantities that are quite independent of the amount of oil in the diet.

For a while there was speculation about the role of the halogen chemicals—iodine, bromine, and fluorine—in acne formation. These chemicals are found in some food-stuffs and in medications. It is true that in rare cases, iodine or bromine has caused acnelike skin reactions, but it is unlikely that the iodine present in a normal diet, or the fluoride found in many toothpastes, can initiate or aggravate acne.

Nevertheless, lingering doubts and long-held dietary prejudices encourage many dermatologists to play it safe and tell their acne patients to avoid the particular foods that they believe aggravate their acne.

Stress and Emotional Factors

There is no doubt whatsoever that acne can create emotional problems for the person who has it. Studies have shown that people with mild acne have much the same psychological profile as people without acne, but people with severe acne have a wide range of mild to severe emotional reactions, including anxiety, depression, anger, and lowered self-esteem. To be sure, part of this emotional reaction is related to our cultural values, which tend to overemphasize the importance of the physical appearance, particularly the skin.

Evidence for the opposite situation, that our emotions can *cause* acne, is much less obvious. There is some suggestion that occasional stress in some individuals can cause acne to flare, as in the case of college students at exam time, but the role of stress in the ups and downs of acne is generally overestimated.

One aspect of the role of the emotions in causing acne is not at all controversial. A condition called acne excoriée (*excoriée* means "scratched or abraded") takes in those acne sufferers who are chronic self-mutilators, compulsively picking and squeezing pimples and damaging their skin far beyond the injury caused by the acne condition itself. The severity of this emotional problem varies. Mild pickers can break the habit themselves when the destruc-

Causes of Acne

tive nature of their behavior is pointed out to them. Severe pickers, on the other hand, who find tiny insignificant blemishes and turn them into large craters and permanent scars, are more difficult to restrain and may require professional counseling.

Despite the fact that currently accepted theories about the origins of acne leave little room for prevention, and long-accepted influences (particularly stress and diet) are more mythical than real, there is no reason for despair. Acne can be treated effectively and controlled, even cured.

3

Treatment: Self-Help

When it comes to self-treatment, remember the old adage a little goes a long way. Family physicians and dermatologists frequently encounter patients with severe skin irritations and rashes from what is commonly referred to as overtreatment. On the other hand, patients rarely seek professional help for their acne without first trying home remedies and over-the-counter medications.

Even if you think your acne can be managed without professional guidance or prescribed medications, you still need correct and up-to-date information on skin hygiene, over-the-counter external medications, nonprescription internal drugs, the pros and cons of removing blackheads or squeezing blemishes, the effects of sunlight and artificial ultraviolet therapy, and the efficacy of the beauty salon approach to acne treatment.

SELF-TREATMENTS

Cleaning the Skin

Since it is generally agreed that clean or dirty skin has little to do with the absence or presence of acne, is there any reason to wash or otherwise regularly clean acne-affected skin as part of a general treatment program? The answer, of course, is yes, but with a caveat: Don't overdo it!

Soap and water remove sebum, bacteria and other microorganisms, and dead cells that accumulate on the skin's surface. The rare individuals who refuse to clean their skin frequently develop irritations or rashes and are more subject to infections. But many more skin problems are associated with overzealous skin hygiene than with neglect.

In the case of acne, you should certainly wash your face in a normal fashion. And for the do-it-yourselfers who want something more than soap and water, there are alternative products.

Medicated Soaps. A number of soaps are available that contain medications (usually benzoyl peroxide) also found in over-the-counter lotions and creams used to treat acne. These preparations clean the skin and leave a deposit of the medication on the skin's surface. Since the concentration of the active ingredient in the soap is generally low and much of it is rinsed away, its effectiveness is limited. Nevertheless, these medicated cleansers can be quite drying, particularly when used in conjunction with other medications that also have drying properties. Some dermatologists favor the use of these medicated soaps to promote drying and peeling. Others prefer to use the same medication in more precise concentrations in the form of a lotion, cream, or gel.

Treatment: Self-Help

MEDICATED SOAPS

Help to keep skin clean and dry up blemishes, but excessive use can result in overdrying of skin. Try using the soap once a day, preferably at night, to gauge your reaction. If your skin tolerates the soap well, use it more often. If you are using other drying medications and ointments at the same time, it's probably best to limit your use of the soap to once a day.

Abrasive Cleansers. Abrasive cleansers contain fine particles such as ground-up fruit pits, aluminum salts, or polyethylene plastic that abrade the skin and eliminate cellular debris and small acne blemishes. A study of the effectiveness of these products showed that they did not eliminate comedones. Most skin specialists, therefore, do not recommend the use of abrasive cleansers. They can damage already weakened follicles, causing breakage of the follicle walls and transforming noninflamed blocked follicles into pimples.

ABRASIVE SOAPS AND CLEANSERS

Not recommended. Regular use of these products can damage already weakened follicles and aggravate the acne condition.

Astringents. Astringents—alcohol-containing lotions that remove oil from the skin and produce a dry, tight sensation—are popular cleansing agents among acne sufferers as well as among people with very oily skin. Astringents are designed to be very drying, and some individuals cannot

TREATING ACNE

tolerate their regular use, particularly if they are used in conjunction with other acne medications that also have drying properties. Since astringents do not alter any of the root causes of acne, it makes more sense to discard them in favor of drying medications that can change the course of acne.

ASTRINGENTS

These products are sometimes useful for removing excess oil from the skin. Employ as a supplement to regular soap and water washing. You may find that the alcohol base causes excessive drying of the skin, so try using the product only once a day at first to ascertain your reaction to it. Do not overuse.

Nonsoap Cleansers. Unlike conventional cold cream or cleansing cream, a group of nonsoap cleansers are available that contain no fatty substances that might block pores or foster the formation of comedones. These so-called lipid-free cleansers come in a liquid form and are used without water. They are of special value for people with acne and dry skin and for do-it-yourselfers who tend to overtreat themselves with drying medications. Dermatologists use these cleansers not only for acne but also in the treatment of eczema and other forms of dermatitis in which dryness contributes to the problem.

NONSOAP CLEANSERS

Helpful for acne sufferers who have an inherently dry skin or dryness resulting from overuse of medications. Use twice a day, morning and evening, in place of regular soap.

Treatment: Self-Help 31

In summary, in acne as in healthy skin, regular cleansing is necessary to remove sebum, bacteria, and dead cells. It is questionable whether cleansing agents are appropriate ways to apply medications that can be applied in a more controlled manner in other forms. It is generally agreed that washing too frequently or too vigorously and using abrasive cleansers can damage already weakened follicles and actually make the acne worse.

Exfoliants

The word *exfoliate* means "to peel." An exfoliant is a substance that, when applied to the skin, promotes scaling and the sloughing off of the topmost layer of cells. Exfoliants work in large part because they cause a minor irritation referred to as "counterirritation," much like oil of wintergreen or other muscle rubs that produce a mild redness and warmth when applied to the skin. In this manner, exfoliants increase blood flow to the skin, which, along with the peeling effect, hastens the resolution of minor acne blemishes, papules, and pustules.

In addition to soap and astringents, exfoliants are among the oldest self-help preparations used to treat acne. These products contain elemental sulfur in various forms, salicylic acid, and resorcinol and are available in prescription and nonprescription acne medications. Some are tinted and act as a cosmetic cover-up as they dry up blemishes. An old standby known as Vleminckx Solution—which some dermatologists still occasionally use to treat severe pustular and cystic acne—contains a sulfur compound.

The major criticism of exfoliants is their failure to treat any of the root causes of acne. With the exception of salicylic acid in relatively high concentrations, which is potentially irritating, exfoliants do not eliminate comedones or open blocked follicles, nor do they decrease sebum excretion or the number of acne bacteria present in the follicles.

Light freezing of the skin with dry ice or liquid nitrogen

TREATING ACNE

is another method that causes exfoliation. It is used by dermatologists in their offices (see Chapter 4).

EXFOLIANTS

If used cautiously, these products can help conceal and dry up blemishes. Apply after cleaning skin. Excessive use can cause further irritation that may resemble an acne flare-up. Follow the instructions on the label for best results.

Benzoyl Peroxide

Perhaps one of the most effective topical medications used to treat acne, benzoyl peroxide is the main active ingredient in some of the most popular over-the-counter acne products and is prescribed in other forms extensively by family physicians and dermatologists. Benzoyl peroxide is available in concentrations of 2.5 percent, 5 percent, and 10 percent in the form of lotions, creams, and gels. It is also an ingredient in some soaps and cleansing lotions.

The primary function of benzoyl peroxide is to kill the acne bacteria inside the follicles and thus reduce the inflammation. In addition to its antibacterial quality, it is a drying agent and functions as an exfoliant. Finally, it has been suggested by some researchers that it may even decrease the amount of oil produced by the sebaceous glands. All in all, it is a very versatile medication and very helpful to acne sufferers.

The major side effect of benzoyl peroxide arises from its drying properties. Even at the lowest concentrations, many users experience excessive peeling and, sometimes, rashes. In addition to dryness, some people are truly allergic to this compound. About 3 percent of the population will develop an allergic rash if they come in contact with

Treatment: Self-Help

benzoyl peroxide in any concentration and in any form. If you know that you are sensitive or allergic to benzoyl peroxide, be sure to check the ingredients listed on any over-the-counter medication you purchase. This is important, since most of the nonprescription acne preparations do not mention benzoyl peroxide in the product's name.

Benzoyl peroxide is often the first self-help treatment you select. If it proves ineffective by itself, it can be used in combination with other prescription medications or as part of an overall program of professional treatment that might include oral medications.

Like hydrogen peroxide, benzoyl peroxide is a bleaching agent. Be careful not to bring this medication into contact with clothing.

BENZOYL PEROXIDE PRODUCTS

Some of the most effective over-the-counter products contain benzoyl peroxide. For mild cases, start with a 2.5-percent concentration and increase, if necessary, to 5 percent, then to 10 percent. Apply once or twice daily. Discontinue immediately if redness, itching, or excessive drying and peeling develop.

Internal Medications

Few if any nonprescription oral medications have been used to treat acne in recent years, yet many people still ask about the value of vitamin supplements in the diet, particularly vitamin A. Since acne is not a vitamin-deficiency disease, such therapy is not helpful or appropriate. In fact, very large doses of vitamin A, such as 300,000 to 500,000 units daily (the daily normal requirement is only 5,000 units), are *not* recommended. Taking large doses of vitamin A can cause numerous side effects because the vitamin accumulates in the body, resulting in dry skin, hair loss, nosebleeds, and, more seriously, neurological problems and liver disease. One good thing that can be said about vitamin A, however, is that an awareness of its positive effects on acne and other skin disorders has led to the development of a group of drugs that are very similar to vitamin A but have fewer side effects.

It is difficult to say why zinc became a popular form of acne treatment several years ago. A deficiency of zinc is rare, perhaps nonexistent, in otherwise healthy people, but when it does occur it results in hair loss and unusual rashes, not acne. In any case, zinc treatment has no effect on acne and has been abandoned. It should be noted, however, that zinc has recently been incorporated into some acne lotions but only because it seems to increase the effectiveness of the antibiotics in these lotions.

At various times other mineral and dietary supplements have been used to treat acne, but no evidence exists that anything you buy in your local health food store will help. Most doctors recommend a well-balanced diet, supplemented by vitamins and minerals only if appropriate for reasons other than the presence of acne.

Self-Surgery

Dermatologists refer to the removal of comedones, the opening of pustules, and the removal of cysts as acne surgery, and there is some disagreement among them as to the value of some of these procedures. Most dermatologists agree that removing blackheads will provide, if nothing else, temporary cosmetic improvement. But do other forms of surgery improve the course of acne and prevent scarring? Some argue yes, others no. No doubt, with the availability of new alternative forms of treatment, fewer and fewer dermatologists will perform acne surgery on a routine basis.

This controversy among professionals should instill a

Treatment: Self-Help   35

sense of caution if you are considering taking matters into
your own hands and performing a little self-surgery. Even
removing blackheads can be harmful if not done properly.
Like removing a splinter, it's not easy to do yourself. The
instrument designed to make it simpler, the comedone extractor, is most effective in the hands of someone who is
experienced in the technique.

Squeezing blemishes is almost always destructive, since
it takes only a little pressure to break the already weakened
wall of the affected follicle and spread the inflammation
into the adjacent tissue. There are pus pimples, sometimes
referred to as whiteheads, where a flaccid, pus-filled pimple sits on top of a reddened area of skin, which will rupture with minimal pressure. But it will also rupture simply
by washing the skin or applying a warm compress, both
of which avoid the potential damage resulting from
squeezing.

Incising a blemish yourself with a needle or a scalpel
blade is also a risky business. It can cause additional injury
to the skin and increase the chance of scar formation. On
the other hand, the use of exfoliants or just leaving minor
blemishes alone until they go away by themselves will not
lead to scarring.

It is inevitable that some people will not be able to resist
the temptation of doing a little self-surgery now and again,
so a few words of caution are in order: The golden rule of
all surgery is to treat tissue gently. Do less rather than
more, and always do it antiseptically. Clean the skin with
alcohol or some other antiseptic both before and after. If
over the ensuing hours or days the treated area gets worse
rather than better, consult a dermatologist.

Emergencies

When a large, angry blemish appears on the nose or the
chin the day before a wedding, prom, or college interview,
it is truly a cosmetic emergency. What to do? The tempta-

TREATING ACNE

tion is to destroy the unsightly thing: squeeze it, pick it, cut it open, anything to get rid of it. Don't! That only makes it worse. There is no quick fix for the emergency blemish, but there are several things you can do to help the situation.

- Hot compresses (don't burn yourself!) using plain water and a soft cloth applied for ten minutes every two to three hours will bring blood and white blood cells into the area and speed the resolution of the pimple.

- In between compresses, apply either a 5-percent benzoyl peroxide gel or one of the over-the-counter sulfur and salicylic acid creams or lotions to promote drying and exfoliation.

- If the blemish remains very red, a few hours before the big event try some cold compresses or an ice cube application to constrict the small blood vessels and temporarily reduce the redness.

- Use a good cover-up makeup stick to hide the residue of the blemish.

- For major emergencies—very large blemishes or very important occasions—consider seeing a dermatologist for additional emergency treatments that may be helpful.

Sunlight and Sunlamps

If you are among the 50 percent of acne sufferers whose acne improves in the summertime, then natural sunlight or some form of artificial ultraviolet light may be a therapeutic option. But again, don't overdo it. You will probably accomplish your goals by staying only an hour or two in the sun; a whole day at the beach can be harmful. Keep in mind that ultraviolet rays are not entirely user friendly. The changes in the skin produced by ultraviolet light are gradual and cumulative, leading inevitably to premature aging, wrinkling, discolorations and benign skin growths, and skin cancer. Use a sun block that provides some protection but does not totally eliminate the therapeutic value of the sun.

Treatment: Self-Help   37

Artificial light delivered by sunlamps and other modern sources of ultraviolet rays is an effective form of treatment for a number of skin diseases, particularly psoriasis. In the case of acne, there are so many other forms of treatment that many dermatologists have abandoned ultraviolet light therapy so as not to inflict sun damage on their acne patients.

Tanning parlors are definitely *not* recommended. These places are not licensed or regulated, and the amount of ultraviolet light delivered at a session is at the whim of the operator. A healthy tan may improve and obscure acne, but other long-term skin changes must be considered. Visiting a tanning parlor before the summer or before a trip to the Caribbean to get your skin in shape for further sun exposure is dangerous, because ultraviolet ray skin damage is additive and cumulative.

Beauty Salons

Many beauty salons offer some forms of acne treatment, including cleansing the skin, removing blackheads, and opening closed comedones and small pustules by trained operators. Often a line of antiacne cosmetics (generally expensive) is sold as part of the overall package. Since these salons are in business to help their clientele, these treatment plans are generally safe, even if not always effective. Occasionally treatments are overdone and clients emerge with an irritated skin from overzealous manipulations and treatments.

Often the treatment consists of a facial, which includes the application of one or more masks designed to provide a deep cleansing of the skin. The mask, usually a mixture of powdery claylike substances with an astringent added, is applied to the face and then washed off after a suitable period of time. For do-it-yourselfers, most cosmetics counters in large department stores carry a line of facial masks designed for treating acne or oily skin. Dermatologists sometimes recommend medicated masks as part of exfoliant therapy.

How effective is the facial performed in the beauty salon? From an aesthetic point of view, a facial can be a pleasant and relaxing experience regardless of the contents and actions of the materials applied to the skin. It is doubtful, however, that it accomplishes more than the ordinary cleansing or the application of exfoliant and astringent medications. Much the same can be said for so-called therapeutic cosmetics. Be aware that cosmetics, unlike medications approved by the Food and Drug Administration (FDA), are not subjected to rigorous testing to prove or disprove claims of efficacy. A "deep cleanser" may not be any more effective in cleaning the pores than ordinary soap and water applied with a clean washcloth.

4

Treatment: Seeing a Dermatologist

Even if your acne is on the mild side, and you believe that you can manage it yourself, there is still something to be said for seeing a doctor, preferably a dermatologist, for a consultation. The dermatologist, who has seen hundreds, if not thousands, of patients with your type of acne, can assess the severity of your problem and indicate the likely prognosis and potential for scarring. He or she can answer questions and offer advice about skin care and appropriate treatment for your type of blemishes.

If your doctor suggests using prescription medications, he or she will probably encourage you to accept continuing care and return for a follow-up appointment. While you may not be inclined to do this, do not expect the doctor to write prescriptions indefinitely. Once the dermatologist has prescribed treatment, he or she cannot be held responsible on a continuing basis without periodically evaluating your response to treatment and adjusting dosages or changing medications if appropriate.

When discussing your treatment, the dermatologist

TREATING ACNE

should explain that medications are slow to take effect. With the exception of exfoliants, which provide immediate cosmetic improvement (they are popular for that reason), most acne-suppressive medications take weeks to months to provide real improvement.

PRESCRIBED ACNE TREATMENTS
Tretinoin (Retin A)

Retin A is an externally applied medication that has recently received considerable attention as an antiwrinkle, anti–sun damage cream. Although it is widely prescribed for these purposes, as of this writing it has not received FDA approval for this use. In contrast, the FDA has found Retin A to be a safe and effective treatment for acne, and for years dermatologists have prescribed it to treat mild to moderately severe acne conditions. (One of the differences in using Retin A for treating sun-damaged skin versus acne is that the medication must be used indefinitely to treat the former while as an acne treatment it is usually applied for a few months to a year or two at the most.)

Retin A is actually *retinoic acid*, a derivative of vitamin A, and is currently the most effective externally applied medication to rid the skin of comedones. Not only does it eliminate existing blackheads and closed comedones, but it also prevents new ones from forming and thus alters the entire process that leads to the development of papules, pustules, and other inflammatory blemishes.

Different forms of Retin A preparations are available—creams, gels, and liquids—in concentrations ranging from .01 percent to 0.1 percent. Since skin irritation, usually redness, dryness, and peeling, is a relatively common side effect, most doctors start treatment with the mildest preparations, the .01 percent gel or the 0.025 percent cream, and increase the strength only if necessary.

Retin A is applied once a day, usually at night. Use small

Treatment: Seeing a Dermatologist 41

quantities and avoid sensitive areas such as the corners of the mouth and nose and the area around the eyes. It is important that your skin be scrupulously dry, since applying the medication to wet skin increases its irritative potential. In order to keep irritation to a minimum, use a mild soap and do not wash the area too often. Furthermore, since Retin A–induced peeling makes the skin more vulnerable to sunburn, apply a sunscreen with an SPF of at least 15 if you intend to spend time in the sun. Some dermatologists recommend not using Retin A at all during the summer months or on other occasions when intense exposure to the sun is likely.

Despite all of these precautions, some degree of stinging, redness, and slight peeling occurs in most people during the early weeks of treatment, but the irritation does subside even though treatment is continued. Your acne may even get worse, and after a month of daily applications there may be a flare-up of new papules and pustules. Don't despair. Believe it or not, this is an encouraging sign, suggesting that the Retin A is working. A few weeks after the flare-up you will see improvement, and it will continue. Many Retin A users abandon the medication prematurely and are reluctant to give it a second chance ("I'm not going through that again"). But this doubt and uncertainty can be avoided if you receive proper instructions before starting treatment.

Except where the outbreak consists of only comedones, Retin A is usually prescribed in conjunction with other medications such as benzoyl peroxide and/or antibiotics. Some evidence suggests that Retin A, because it peels and thins the skin, actually increases the penetration and effectiveness of the other applied medications.

Topical Antibiotics

Although oral antibiotics have been known since the 1950s to be effective in treating acne, it wasn't until twenty-five

TREATING ACNE

years later that topical, or externally applied, antibiotics came into use. In retrospect it seems likely that the potential value of topical antibiotics was neglected because it was thought that the medication would not penetrate the skin deeply enough to reach the bacteria. In 1978 it was demonstrated that, with the proper delivery system, topical antibiotics did work.

Externally applied antibiotics penetrate into the follicles and kill or reduce the bacteria that are so important in the development of papules, pustules, and cysts. Several antibiotics currently in use—erythromycin, clindamycin, tetracycline, and meclocycline—provide good results. Erythromycin and clindamycin are equally effective and are the most popular of these preparations. They are formulated as water-and-alcohol solutions, creamy lotions, gels, and, in the case of erythromycin, as an ointment. When applied twice a day to mild or moderately severe acne with predominantly papules and pustules, some improvement may be seen in as little as two weeks. In most cases, however, maximum improvement requires eight to twelve weeks. Comparative studies suggest that topical antibiotics are as effective as oral tetracycline in reducing papules and pustules.

The major advantage of topical over oral antibiotics is the absence of side effects. In fact, side effects from topical antibiotics are infrequent and rarely severe. Dryness, peeling, and itching are usually due to the alcohol in the solution, not the antibiotic itself. Allergic reactions, in the form of a rash, are rare.

In theory, when bacteria are exposed to an antibiotic day after day, the bacteria can develop a resistance to the point where the antibiotic loses its effectiveness and no longer suppresses or kills the bacteria. This is a rare problem in acne treatment. When it does happen, and the antibiotic is discontinued, susceptible strains of the bacteria quickly return and the same antibiotic becomes effective again. But generally it isn't necessary to discontinue antibiotic therapy altogether, since a variety of other classes of antibiotics

Treatment: Seeing a Dermatologist

are available that are likely to be active against the resistant bacteria.

Far more common is a less well defined form of antibiotic resistance. After months, sometimes years, of continued and successful use of the same antibiotic, many new blemishes suddenly start to appear even while the antibiotic is still being used. The new outbreak often responds to a change in antibiotic, even to one that is similar to the original medication. Why antibiotics lose their effectiveness in this way after prolonged use is not entirely clear.

Topical antibiotics can be used with other medications, both external and internal. Antibiotics and benzoyl peroxide are a popular combination, for example. In fact, there is an erythromycin–benzoyl peroxide all-in-one preparation that is nonirritating and seems to be more effective than using either medication by itself. Topical antibiotics and Retin A are also used together, although not in the same preparation.

Since most of the topical antibiotic preparations get the job done, the decision about which to use is often based on other considerations. Costs vary, but since competition in the marketplace is stiff—there are many preparations to choose from—prices fall within a relatively narrow range. The types of preparations formulated by the manufacturers can differ—some feel sticky, others may seem too drying or too greasy. To some people, convenience of application is important. Lotion bottles come equipped with special applicators and delivery systems, and antibiotic-impregnated pledgettes (disposable pads) are handy for application away from home. Finally, if excessive drying is a problem, as it often is when other drying medications are also being used, mildly moisturizing erythromycin ointment or meclocycline cream may be the better choice.

Oral Antibiotics

Although oral antibiotics are usually no more effective than topical antibiotics for mild to moderately severe acne,

TREATING ACNE

they are almost a necessity for treating severe acne in which there are deep papules, large pustules, and cysts. Often oral antibiotics are used in conjunction with topical antibiotics or other externally applied medications. The treatment plan is to bring the acne under control with the combination of oral and topical medications, wean the patient from the oral antibiotic, and then try to maintain the improvement using topical medications alone. All this is done over a period of months, since maximum improvement takes upward of three to four months with oral antibiotics.

Tetracycline. Tetracycline, the first oral antibiotic to be used to treat acne, is still the favorite of most dermatologists because it is effective, safe, and relatively inexpensive. Most patients are started on a dose of 1 gram daily, 250 milligrams four times a day, or 500 milligrams twice a day. You take the pills on an empty stomach, one hour before or two hours after eating, since food, particularly dairy products, interferes with its absorption into the body. If you experience nausea from taking tetracycline before eating, it is still effective if taken one half hour after eating or even with a small amount of food (not a milk product). Once absorbed into the body, tetracycline gets into the bloodstream and is carried to the skin, where it acts on the acne bacteria in the same way topical antibiotics do.

Side effects from tetracycline are sometimes a problem. Women on long-term tetracycline therapy may develop a vaginal infection due to the yeast fungus *Candida albicans*. This fungus occurs because the tetracycline eliminates bacteria from the intestine. Under normal circumstances, these bacteria compete with yeast organisms and keep the yeast population in the intestine from expanding. With their removal, yeast organisms proliferate and make their way to the outside and into the vagina. This problem can be avoided (or treated) to some extent by taking Nystatin, an antiyeast antibiotic, along with the tetracycline. It is

Treatment: Seeing a Dermatologist   45

also helpful to eat yogurt (not frozen) or some other source of the bacteria that normally inhabit the intestinal tract. Some women are prone to recurrent yeast infections and therefore are not good candidates for prolonged antibiotic therapy. The majority of women, however, can take antibiotics without experiencing this unpleasant side effect.

Other side effects may include stomach upset and irritation of the esophagus, which can make swallowing painful. Some tetracycline takers also experience sun sensitivity and either sunburn more easily or develop a rash when exposed to the sun. Limiting sun exposure and using a sun block usually prevent this problem. Tetracycline cannot be used by young children or pregnant or nursing women, since it can affect developing teeth and bones and cause permanent yellowish discoloration of the teeth.

Tetracycline and some of the other antibiotics may also decrease the effectiveness of birth control pills. For that reason, it's prudent to use a backup form of contraception while taking tetracycline.

The potential side effects of tetracycline may sound formidable, but, with the exception of tooth discoloration, they are all reversible with discontinuation of the medication. Considering the amount of tetracycline prescribed for acne, side effects requiring discontinuation of this medication are rare.

Other Antibiotics. The other antibiotics used to treat acne are erythromycin, minocycline, doxycycline, and a combination drug, trimethoprim sulfamethoxazole. Erythromycin is an excellent second choice if tetracycline doesn't produce the desired effects or if it can't be tolerated because of a side effect. It is the first choice for treating younger children because it does not affect developing teeth and bones. However, upset stomach, cramps, and diarrhea are more common with erythromycin than tetracycline, and these unpleasant symptoms are the main reason that this medication may have to be discontinued.

TREATING ACNE

To some extent these gastrointestinal side effects can be avoided by taking erythromycin with food or by using one of the newer, coated tablets that are less irritating to the intestine. Erythromycin is safe to take during pregnancy, although topical treatment of acne is preferable during this time.

Minocycline and doxycycline are derivatives of tetracycline. Minocycline, which is particularly popular in treating acne, is considered by many doctors to be the most effective antibiotic for that purpose. It is, however, rarely the first choice for treatment because it is much more expensive than either tetracycline or erythromycin. A short course of minocycline is a tolerable expense, but if it has to be taken for months, the treatment can break the family budget. Minocycline can cause many of the same side effects as tetracycline, but stomach and intestinal complaints are less frequent. Unlike tetracycline, patients taking minocycline sometimes experience dizziness or a lightheaded sensation, which can usually be alleviated by reducing the dose. A rare side effect—a muddy discoloration of the skin—occurs in individuals who have been taking minocycline for many months to a period of years. As in the case of most medications, minocycline can cause allergic reactions of the skin, particularly hives. Sun sensitivity can occur with minocycline and doxycycline but less frequently than it does with tetracycline.

A rare complication of long-term oral antibiotic treatment of acne is the occurrence of a true pustular infection of the skin. This arises in a manner similar to the development of the yeast infection associated with tetracycline. Bacteria that are not suppressed or killed by the tetracycline or erythromycin flourish and cause an infection of the follicles. This complication is heralded by the abrupt flare-up of otherwise well controlled acne, with many small pustules appearing all over the face. Fortunately, there are other antibacterial medications, such as some of the sulfa drugs and forms of penicillin, that can eliminate this type of infection.

Treatment: Seeing a Dermatologist 47

Over the years there has been considerable concern that the long-term treatment of acne with oral antibiotics would make adolescents and young adults susceptible to other infections that might not respond to antibiotic treatment. Forty years' experience with tetracycline has reassured doctors that respiratory and other infections do not occur with greater frequency among individuals on long-term antibiotic treatment, nor are they any more difficult to treat when they do occur. Furthermore, time and experience have shown that there are no long-term side effects from taking antibiotics for even long periods of time.

Hormones

Estrogens. It is well known that androgens (male hormones) increase the size and oil production of the sebaceous glands and thus contribute to the development of acne. Treatment to counter the action of androgens became popular in the 1960s with the advent of the birth control pill. It is the estrogen (female hormone) portion of the pill that reduces sebum production and improves acne. The early birth control pills, which contained relatively large amounts of estrogen, were particularly effective in treating acne. But the side effects of the pill—nausea, weight gain, breast tenderness, spotting, and the risk of phlebitis and other blood vessel problems—caused the amount of estrogen in the pill to be decreased. Although just as effective for contraceptive purposes, the currently prescribed pill is not as effective in treating acne as the original pill. Nevertheless, birth control pills that contain 30 micrograms of ethinyl estradiol (estrogen) can be appropriate for young women whose acne is not responsive to other forms of treatment. (Birth control pills cannot be used in males with acne because they have feminizing side effects, such as breast enlargement.) It takes two or three cycles of the pill for any noticeable improvement, so a little patience is required.

48   TREATING ACNE

The action of birth control pills on the oil glands becomes all too evident when women discontinue their use. The abrupt withdrawal of the estrogen results in an increase in oil gland activity and, in some instances, the appearance of acne in women who never previously had a skin problem. In most cases, estrogen withdrawal acne will resolve itself after a few months.

Some women cannot take birth control pills because of an existing illness or a predisposition to an illness such as inflammation of the veins (phlebitis), migraine headaches, heart disease, depression, or cancer. Also, women who are heavy smokers or who have high blood pressure are not good candidates for the pills.

Antiandrogens. There are other medications that block the action of androgens on the oil glands and thus help improve an acne condition. These drugs, called antiandrogens, are more widely used in Europe to treat acne than in the United States. Spironolactone, a drug designed to treat high blood pressure and some heart-related problems, has also been used to treat acne in women because it has antiandrogen properties. Side effects include dizziness, fatigue, nausea, and often a disturbance of the menstrual cycle. Like the birth control pill, spironolactone cannot be prescribed for males because of its feminizing effects. The other antiandrogen that is widely used in Great Britain but has not yet been approved for use in the United States is cyproterone. Used in combination with estrogen, cyproterone is an effective antiacne birth control pill. Side effects are said to be relatively infrequent.

It has been suggested that acne sufferers are different from people without acne because they have oil glands that are unusually sensitive to normal amounts of androgens. There are, however, individuals with acne, mostly women, who are overproducing these hormones in the ovaries or the adrenal glands. In addition to the acne, some of these women also have irregular menstrual periods and an in-

Treatment: Seeing a Dermatologist 49

crease in body hair. Special tests can determine if the excess androgens are coming from the ovaries or from the adrenal glands. If the ovaries are the source of the excessive androgen production, the treatment is determined by the nature of the ovarian abnormality. It may include surgery or treatment with estrogen or other hormones.

If the adrenal glands are the source of the excess androgens, they can be "turned off" by giving small doses of corticosteroids (cortisonelike drugs). The acne condition improves after several months. Unfortunately there can be problems in taking even small doses of corticosteroids over a prolonged period of time. These include fluid retention and weight gain, stretch marks, and a rise in blood pressure.

Corticosteroids are used to treat acne not only because they turn off adrenal androgen production but also because of their so-called anti-inflammatory effects. These same medications are used in all areas of medicine to treat many forms of inflammation. In acne, corticosteroids are prescribed for brief periods to treat severe inflammations that are not responding to other medications. But because of the side effects and the advent of Accutane (discussed below), they are used less and less frequently.

In addition to taking corticosteroids by mouth, there is another safe and very effective way of administering this medication. Using a syringe and a very fine needle, a dermatologist can inject small amounts of diluted corticosteroid directly into large blemishes and inflammatory cysts. This relatively painless procedure results in rapid improvement of the area, sometimes complete elimination of the blemish within a few days. A dermatologist can treat the serious emergency pimple in this way. This intralesional injection is the dermatologist's "magic bullet." Since the dose of corticosteroid is very small, there is no risk of side effects that might occur with taking corticosteroid orally. Occasionally, injecting corticosteroid causes a depression in the skin at that area, which may take several

TREATING ACNE

months to fill in. This is the only adverse effect that has been seen using this procedure.

Accutane

Accutane, the trade name for isotretinoin, has been described as the greatest single advance in the treatment of acne. Certainly not since the 1960s, when antibiotics were first used, has a drug come along that has so improved the prognosis for patients suffering the most serious forms of inflammatory, potentially scarring, cystic acne. Accutane, like its cousin Retin A (tretinoin), is closely related to vitamin A. But unlike vitamin A, which can cause a lot of side effects because it builds up in the body to toxic levels, Accutane is rapidly broken down in the body and excreted. This is not to say that Accutane does not have side effects—it most certainly does—but it can be used to treat acne whereas vitamin A cannot.

How does Accutane work? Nobody knows for sure. The medication's most obvious action is on the oil glands, which become smaller and manufacture far less sebum than do normal oil glands. Because of potentially serious side effects, Accutane is recommended only if you have severe acne with large papules and cysts that do not respond to other forms of treatment.

A course of treatment with Accutane lasts sixteen to twenty weeks. The medication is taken by mouth in doses that are determined by your weight. It takes four to eight weeks for any improvement to become noticeable, and there is commonly a flare-up of the acne before sustained improvement occurs. One of the striking things about Accutane is that improvement may continue for weeks to months after a course of treatment has been completed and despite the fact that all of the medication has left the body.

Almost 90 percent of Accutane users show improvement, an incredible statistic compared to other forms of

Treatment: Seeing a Dermatologist

treatment. And almost half of Accutane-treated acne clears completely and requires no further treatment, although a small number of significantly improved patients relapse and a second course of treatment may be necessary.

If Accutane is such a remarkable drug, why not give it to everyone with acne? Because there are a number of potential side effects. The mildest is related to the action of Accutane on the oil glands. Foremost are dry skin with itching and rash, chapped lips, dryness inside the nose that sometimes results in nosebleeds, and various forms of eye irritation. Almost everyone who takes Accutane experiences some of these symptoms, but they are made manageable by using lubricants and skin lotions and rarely lead to discontinuation of the treatment. Some Accutane users experience aches and pains in bones, muscles, and joints. Again, these symptoms are rarely severe enough to stop treatment, and they disappear shortly after a course of treatment is completed.

Other, more serious side effects occur less frequently but may be reasons to discontinue the medication. These include changes in liver function as determined by blood tests, elevation of cholesterol and triglycerides (fatty substances) in the blood, and headaches due to increased pressure inside the skull.

Potentially the most serious side effect can occur in pregnant women. In the early stages of pregnancy, Accutane can affect the development of the fetus and result in miscarriage, stillbirth, and serious birth defects and malformations. Because of this, doctors should perform a pregnancy test on any female of childbearing age before starting a course of treatment with Accutane. Furthermore, they are advised to instruct female patients on appropriate methods of contraception. Bear in mind, however, that the effects of Accutane are not lasting. Once treatment with Accutane is completed and the user experiences a normal menstrual cycle, it is safe to become pregnant without risk of Accutane-induced fetal abnormalities.

TREATING ACNE

Because of these potential side effects, your doctor must monitor you closely if you choose to use the drug. In addition to pretreatment pregnancy testing, other blood tests before and during treatment are necessary, particularly to check on liver function, cholesterol, and serum triglycerides. As you can see, embarking on a course of treatment with Accutane is a serious proposition that requires discipline and commitment on your part and your doctor's diligence. Unlike some other forms of treatment, a little Accutane is of no value; a full sixteen- to twenty-week course of treatment is necessary to realize the full benefits of this unusual drug.

NAME	WHAT IT DOES	POSSIBLE SIDE EFFECTS
Tretinoin (Retin A)	Eliminates and prevents comedones	Dryness, redness, peeling, sun sensitivity
Topical antibiotics (clindamycin, tetracycline, erythromycin, meclocycline)	Destroys acne bacteria	Rarely, dryness or peeling
Oral antibiotics (tetracycline, doxycycline, minocycline)	Destroys acne bacteria	Gastrointestinal upset, swallowing discomfort, vaginal yeast infection, sun sensitivity
Erythromycin	Destroys acne bacteria	Gastrointestinal upset
Hormones— estrogens (including birth control pills)	Decrease size and activity of sebaceous glands	Multiple possible side effects, including weight gain, nausea, mood change, and blood vessel problems

Treatment: Seeing a Dermatologist

Spironolactone	Blocks androgen stimulation of sebaceous glands	Dizziness, fatigue, nausea, irregular menses
Corticosteroids	Reduce skin inflammation	Injected into acne cysts: occasional depression of skin at injection site Systemic—weight gain, blood pressure elevation, mood change, adrenal gland changes
Accutane	Decreases size and activity of sebaceous glands	Multiple—including dry skin, liver and bone problems, and birth defects

Physical Therapy

There are a number of physical procedures that dermatologists may perform on patients with acne. The most widely used methods include cryotherapy (freezing the skin), ultraviolet light therapy, X-ray treatments, and acne surgery.

Cryotherapy. Freezing the skin is a simple and effective treatment, particularly for the pustular and cystic forms of acne. Actually a form of exfoliant therapy, a light freeze provides sufficient irritation of the skin to cause therapeutic peeling.

The dermatologist applies dry ice or a mixture of powdered dry ice and acetone (referred to as "slush") or another, colder freezing agent, liquid nitrogen. The agent is applied briefly, in a matter of seconds, with a cotton swab, a special spray-on apparatus, or a roll-on instrument called a cryoroller. There is mild discomfort, but anesthesia is not required, since the freezing process itself numbs the skin.

After a few days, the skin reddens and peels. To some extent the redness masks the blemishes and the peeling eliminates the papules, pustules, and small cysts. Some physicians favor cryotherapy over the injection of corticosteroids for the treatment of acne cysts. Improvement following cryotherapy is short-lived, but it is a simple, inexpensive form of therapy and therefore popular with patients.

Cryotherapy is also used to treat keloids, the thick, disfiguring scars that appear on the chest and back of some acne patients. In this case the freeze is more vigorous and may have to be repeated several times before the scar flattens out.

Since cryotherapy can sometimes lead to a loss of normal skin pigment, it is not usually recommended for dark-skinned individuals.

X-ray Therapy. Before the introduction of antibiotics in the treatment of acne, the use of X rays was the only effective treatment doctors had to combat the underlying acne process. Superficial X rays, those that do not penetrate deep into the tissue, temporarily reduce the size of the oil glands and markedly decrease the amount of sebum.

In cases of severe acne, a course of X-ray treatments did turn off the acne process as effectively as Accutane does today, but there was a price to pay. Years after X-ray therapy, many individuals who received the radiation had permanently dry, sensitive skin and a tendency to develop skin cancers. Evidence also exists to suggest an increase in cancer of the thyroid gland among adolescents who received X-ray treatment for their acne.

Although a few dermatologists still treat their severe acne patients with superficial X ray, by and large this form of treatment has been replaced by the use of antibiotics, hormonal therapy, and Accutane.

Acne Surgery. The term *acne surgery* refers to a group of simple procedures available to dermatologists to treat se-

Treatment: Seeing a Dermatologist   55

vere acne. These include removing blackheads and whiteheads, opening up small pustules and larger inflammatory
cysts, and incising and emptying tiny white cysts called
"milia."

The surgical methods used routinely by some dermatologists in their offices, as well as by some cosmetologists in
their salons, are described here. It is important to understand that these techniques are by no means endorsed by
all dermatologists. Some believe that these surgical procedures improve the course of acne and prevent scarring;
others believe they only aggravate the condition and increase the chances of scarring. As stated earlier, this controversy should be a warning to potential do-it-yourselfers
that the manipulation of acne blemishes carries certain
risks and should not be undertaken lightly.

Removing Comedones and Milia. There are two different
types of comedones: the open comedone or blackhead,
which represents a blocked pore on the skin surface; and
the closed comedone or whitehead, in which the blockage
exists deeper in the follicle and may lead to the formation
of an inflammatory blemish. The blackhead can be easily
removed with an instrument called a comedone extractor.
These instruments come in different sizes and shapes, but
the basic configuration is a small metal wand with a loop
or opening that is placed over the blocked pore. Pressure
is applied around the opening of the blocked pore, and it
effectively dislodges the comedone. If done properly, there
is no damage to the follicle; if done improperly, the wall of
the follicle can be broken and cause an inflammatory lesion. Some dermatologists or their assistants perform comedone extraction in the office. Rarely do they instruct a
family member in the technique for home care.

Since blackheads are not the source of the inflammatory
lesions of acne, the reason for their removal is immediate
cosmetic improvement. In contrast, eliminating closed
comedones, or whiteheads, removes the blockage of the

duct that is the source of future papules and pustules. Closed comedones, however, are more difficult to deal with. They appear as small whitish bulges on the skin surface. In order to remove the plug, it is necessary to puncture the top of the bulge, thus opening the follicle. Even then it is often difficult to express the plug, and damage from the incision and pressure to expel the contents can be greater than the potential gain. To a great extent the opening of closed comedones has been superseded by the use of Retin A, which eliminates existing comedones and interferes with their formation.

Milia are small whitish cysts that develop not only in acne but also in conjunction with skin injuries and healing wounds. If necessary, they can be managed in the same way as closed comedones—punctured and the seedlike contents of the cyst removed.

Draining Pustules. Even more controversial is the incision and drainage of pustules, pus-filled pimples. The technique involves making a small incision with a pointed scalpel blade and gently pushing out the pus through the incision opening. The procedure hastens the resolution of the pustule, but a scar may form at the incision site. In large pustules the resulting scar may be deep and of the "ice pick" variety, and difficult to eliminate through dermabrasion (see Chapter 6).

Draining Inflammatory Cysts. Cysts are the blemishes that lead to most acne scarring if left untreated. In the past, large cysts were often treated by incision and drainage, thus risking a small scar in the hope of avoiding a large one. Occasionally this method is still necessary for large cysts that are on the verge of rupturing. More often, isolated acne cysts are successfully treated by injecting them with a corticosteroid as described earlier. In the case of severe cystic acne, where multiple cysts form and continue to form, Accutane may be the appropriate treatment.

Acne Treatment During Pregnancy

Many women with acne find that their skin problems improve during pregnancy. This can be explained in part by an increase in estrogen, which acts on the sebaceous glands and decreases the output of sebum. Other women find that pregnancy is not beneficial to their skin, and a small percentage find that their acne is now worse.

In selecting medications to treat acne during pregnancy, safety for mother and fetus is the primary, perhaps the only, consideration. In general, oral medications are avoided even if the acne is not effectively controlled by externally applied medications. In rare circumstances where pustular and cystic acne flares dramatically, a course of erythromycin, an antibiotic safe for both mother and fetus, may be considered.

The externally applied medications discussed here and in previous chapters are considered safe. Even Retin A, a topical medication that is similar to Accutane (a drug known to adversely affect the developing fetus), has been carefully studied and shown to be safe since virtually none of it is absorbed through the skin. Many women prefer to forgo all forms of acne treatment until after birth, but in extreme cases topical erythromycin lotion used in combination with some form of exfoliant therapy is a conservative and safe therapeutic approach.

MILD TO MODERATE ACNE
Medicated cleansers
Exfoliants
Benzoyl peroxide
Retin A
Topical antibiotics
Physical treatments

MODERATE TO SEVERE ACNE

Medicated cleansers

Exfoliants

Benzoyl peroxide

Retin A

Topical antibiotics

Physical treatments

Oral antibiotics

Intralesional
corticosteroids

Hormonal therapy

VERY SEVERE AND CYSTIC ACNE

Medicated cleansers

Exfoliants

Retin A

Topical antibiotics

Physical treatments

Oral antibiotics

Intralesional
corticosteroids

Hormonal therapy

Systemic corticosteroids

Accutane

5

Cosmetics

According to the legal definition, cosmetics are substances that, when applied to the skin, alter the appearance for the better, thus promoting attractiveness. In contrast to medications, cosmetics can make no claim to alter either the function of the skin or to change its structure in any way. Some topical preparations, such as sunscreens, are a combination of cosmetic and medication, but most of the substances we put on our skin are either one or the other.

This distinction between cosmetic and medication is important because the laws and regulations that apply to them differ considerably. Medications are tightly regulated by the Food and Drug Administration (FDA) and are subject to rigorous testing to prove both effectiveness and safety. Furthermore, many aspects of the manufacture of medications are closely scrutinized by the FDA. In short, the public is protected against errors in the manufacturing or labeling of drugs.

In contrast, the cosmetics industry is very loosely regulated. It is assumed, to some extent incorrectly, that cosmetics can do no harm since they do not affect function or alter structure. Consequently the cosmetics industry is not officially obliged to test their products for safety, or to prove their claims about what their cosmetics do when applied to the skin. They are not even required to list all the ingredients on the label if they wish to claim that some of the contents are trade secrets.

In actuality, though, the major manufacturers of cosmetics are very careful about producing uniform, safe, well-labeled products. In an industry as highly competitive as the cosmetics industry, it is essential for survival to produce a reputable product. Reactions to a "bad" cosmetic can trigger costly lawsuits and decrease confidence in the company's other products.

Individuals who are acne-prone or are experiencing a bad case of acne are particularly interested in cosmetics. They want to know which ones aggravate or induce acne, which ones are safe for them to use—and which, if any, have a therapeutic value in an acne situation.

COSMETICS THAT AGGRAVATE ACNE

Some cosmetics cause an almost immediate reaction due to direct irritation of the skin or blockage of the follicle opening. Such preparations are considered acnegenic— that is, tending to cause acne. Shortly after use, papules and small pustules appear in the area where the cosmetic has been applied. One might argue that this is an acnelike eruption rather than a case of true acne, since it resolves rapidly with little treatment once the offending cosmetic has been eliminated.

A more classic form of acne is caused by cosmetics that contain chemicals or oils that initiate the formation of comedones, or blemishes. The concept of comedogenesis, or causing the formation of comedones, has been eagerly taken up by the cosmetics industry in their efforts to create cosmetics that do not cause or aggravate acne. Since the 1950s the comedogenic potential of cosmetics has been studied using what has been called the "rabbit ear" test.

Cosmetics

It was recognized early on that substances applied to a rabbit's ear can cause the formation of comedones in a manner comparable to human comedogenesis. In rabbits the reaction becomes apparent in two weeks of applications, whereas on human skin comedones might not become apparent until after months of repeated applications. For this reason, plus the fact that rabbit volunteers are easier to come by than human subjects, rabbit-ear testing has become the standard industry method of measuring comedogenicity.

Considerable controversy exists regarding the validity of rabbit-ear testing. Many experts feel that it is too sensitive a test, leading to the mislabeling of chemicals as comedogenic that are not likely to cause skin problems in humans. Others feel that the test is not sensitive enough and is difficult to interpret, pointing out the obvious fact that rabbit skin is different from human skin. Nevertheless, there seems to be sufficient correlation between rabbit-ear response and human skin reaction for the cosmetics industry to continue to use this test to create their noncomedogenic cosmetics.

When it comes to the comedogenic potential of various substances, it is not necessarily the degree of oiliness that determines if the material is comedogenic. For example, cocoa butter and coconut oil are very comedogenic, olive oil and peanut oil are only moderately so, and sunflower and safflower oils rate even lower on the comedogenicity scale. Some oils, such as mineral oil, are comedogenic or noncomedogenic depending on their source or how they have been chemically treated. This is also true of lanolin. Acetylated lanolin is very comedogenic, anhydrous lanolin and lanolin alcohol less so, while lanolin oil is considered noncomedogenic.

For those people who are willing to study the labels of cosmetic products before making a purchase, the box on page 62 lists most of the oils and chemicals found in cosmetic preparations that are considered comedogenic. A cosmetic containing one or more of the substances on this list is not recommended for acne-prone individuals.

COMEDOGENIC SUBSTANCES	
Isopropyl myristate	Sodium lauryl sulfate
Myristyl myristate	D&C red dyes 9 and 27
Isopropyl isostearate	Propylene glycol monostearate
Stearic acid	
Glyceryl stearate	Cocoa butter
Butyl stearate	Coconut oil
Isopropyl palmitate	Acetylated lanolin
Decyl oleate	Petrolatum

Unfortunately, the array of labeling claims on cosmetics may be confusing for the customer seeking the best—or the least harmful—products for her skin. For example, some cosmetics may aggravate acne without being comedogenic. These products are considered acnegenic. A number of products are labeled noncomedogenic and others nonacnegenic; the latter is a more inclusive claim. There are "oil-free" and "water-based" cosmetics, but these might still be comedogenic or acnegenic depending on their ingredients. When it comes right down to it, reading labels *is* helpful, but ultimately using the product for an extended period of time is the best way of assessing the cosmetic's ability to cause or aggravate acne.

SELECTING THE BEST COSMETICS FOR YOUR SKIN

Moisturizers

Many women, either out of habit or because of advertising claims, feel that it is essential to use a moisturizer every

Cosmetics 63

day. Since healthy skin makes its own moisturizer, such general use is unwarranted. The notion that moisturizers keep skin youthful-looking and prevent wrinkles is also untrue. Moisturizers are of value only in treating dry skin, which in most cases is related to environmental factors, such as the effects of central heating in the winter or an excessively dry climate.

Moisturizers become an issue for acne sufferers because many of the medications used in treatment are drying, including Retin A, antibiotics in alcohol, benzoyl peroxide, and astringents. Some dermatologists even prefer to modify treatment to prevent excessive drying rather than have a patient routinely use moisturizers that might lead to the formation of more comedones. However, some of the pharmaceutical companies that market acne medications also market moisturizers that are considered safe for people with acne, and an array of comparable dry-skin products are on the market.

Foundations and Powder

Foundations are pigmented cosmetics that lend a uniform color to the skin and mask imperfections such as blemishes and discolorations. Unfortunately the ideal foundation in terms of its ability to conceal and also remain on the skin for an extended period of time is the oil-in-water emulsion, which consists of oil with very little water. For acne-prone individuals with oily skin, it's preferable to use the water-based foundations, which are made up largely of water with only a small amount of added oil.

Cosmeticians recommend applying foundation with a porous cosmetic sponge rather than using a brush or fingertips to produce uniform coverage. After application, the foundation can be "fixed" and enhanced by applying powder. Loose powder is preferable to pressed powder, since the latter contains oil (sometimes mineral oil or isopropyl myristate), which can be comedogenic. Loose powder also absorbs skin oil better than pressed powder, an advantage for oily-skinned users. Powder is most effective if it is massaged into the foundation rather than patted on. Skin-colored powder by itself is often a good cover-up as well.

Blushes

Blush is marketed in liquid, cream, or powder form. Powder blush is the form that acne-prone users should select, since it is not likely to cause comedones or blemishes. Some of the D & C Red pigments are comedogenic, so avoid blushes that are colored with these pigments.

Many blushes, like other cosmetics, do not have their ingredients listed on the container. But persistent use of a comedogenic blush will eventually result in the telltale appearance of acne blemishes concentrated on the cheeks.

Lipstick and Eye Makeup

Lipstick and eye makeup are not likely to aggravate acne, since they are applied to areas of the skin that generally do not develop comedones or acne blemishes. Nevertheless it is reasonable to select eye shadow in powder form rather than one that is oil-based.

TECHNIQUES FOR COVERING ACNE BLEMISHES

Covering up acne blemishes is accomplished by applying foundation and powder in combination or by using either one alone. Since it is the beige or skin-colored pigment in the foundation or powder that masks the redness of acne, sometimes selecting a darker shade of foundation gives better coverage. Multiple applications—that is, layering the foundation—is another maneuver to enhance coverage, but many women justifiably object to the "made up" look that too much foundation creates. You can avoid this by applying the foundation only to the worst areas of red-

Cosmetics

ness and blemishes, allowing it to dry, then applying foundation over the entire face.

Primers, cosmetic preparations that can be used under foundation, also increase coverage. Primers, which use color to hide other color abnormalities, are based on what are called color opposites: blue is the opposite of orange, green the opposite of red, and yellow the opposite of purple. According to this principle, a yellow primer would be most effective in covering up a purplish bruise or birthmark. In the case of acne, a green-tinted primer can be used under the foundation to mask the redness of inflamed skin. In addition to the camouflage effect, primer decreases the amount of foundation needed for effective coverage.

There are other products on the market that are popular for concealing blemishes. Makeup sticks, for example, offer easy application for individual lesions. However, some of these are oil-in-water emulsions, and although they give good coverage, they may be acnegenic. If you prefer not to make up your skin and simply want some basic color coverage, try the brown-colored gels used to simulate a suntan. They provide the cosmetic improvement of tanning without the associated risks.

COSMETIC-MEDICATION COMBINATIONS

As mentioned earlier, some products created by both cosmetics and pharmaceutical companies combine the dual roles of cosmetic and medication. Some of these are medicated cosmetics, others are truly medications, but both are suitable as an acne cover-up.

Cosmetic products used to clean the skin—soaps, cleansing lotions, and abrasive cleaners—sometimes incorporate medications such as benzoyl peroxide or salicylic acid. Although popular, their value is doubtful (see Chapter 3).

Astringents, an acceptable form of treatment for oily skin and mild acne, are marketed by cosmetics companies as oil-control lotions or skin toners. The implication that they control the production of oil is misleading. They do *remove* oil from the skin, as do soap and water, but they do not alter the activity of the oil glands or, for that matter, attack any of the causes of acne. Astringents are marketed as pledgettes—alcohol pads sometimes with salicylic acid added—a convenient way of using the product during the day when you are away from home.

Many medications that have cosmetic potential incorporate benzoyl peroxide, sulfur, salicylic acid or resorcinol, or some combination of these chemicals in a tinted cream or lotion. A few are prescription medicines, but most are available over the counter. Unfortunately, many of the old favorites in this category of drying lotions are being gradually replaced by newer drugs, such as the topical antibiotics, Retin A, and nontinted benzoyl peroxide lotions and gels.

The importance of cosmetics in the treatment of acne should not be minimized. Proper cosmetics, skillfully applied, can alleviate the embarrassment of acne blemishes. Selection of the right cosmetics is important, but equally important is using them to their best advantage. The cosmetics counters of large department stores often offer free lessons in makeup application; it's worthwhile to get their advice if it helps you feel more confident about your appearance.

6

Repairing the Damage: Scars

If your acne is serious enough to warrant medical attention, you may also be wondering if your condition will cause permanent scars. Unfortunately there is no definite yes or no answer, since scarring is dependent on several factors, not all predictable. Certainly the kind of acne lesion you are experiencing is important. Cysts and deep inflammatory papules are more likely to lead to scarring than are comedones, small papules, and superficial pustules. The other less predictable variables are (1) your response to treatment and (2) your skin's tendency to scar from an injury. Sometimes scarring has already occurred before adequate treatment has been started; in other cases, scarring develops despite what seem like adequate measures to prevent it.

The methods that are currently available to treat acne scars include dermabrasion, chemical peels, surgical excision of scars, and the filling in of scars with injections of collagen or other substances. Since these techniques have their pros and cons, it is important for you to become ac-

TREATING ACNE

quainted with the benefits and risks involved in each method. First, though, you should give nature a chance before opting for scar therapy. It is recommended that you wait at least a year from the time that the acne becomes inactive or well controlled by therapy before embarking on one of the scar treatment methods. You may find you don't really need it, thus saving yourself much discomfort, time, and perhaps a considerable outlay of money.

Many of these procedures are costly because they require specialized skills on the part of the operator, considerable input of the operator's time, and sometimes the use of expensive materials. Unfortunately, too, many medical insurers will not provide coverage for plastic or cosmetic surgery, since it is considered an optional procedure rather than necessary medical care. If you are a prospective candidate for one of these procedures, you must determine if your insurance carrier will cover the costs involved. If there is no insurance coverage and you must bear the entire cost, you may elect not to have the procedure performed.

TREATING SCARS

Dermabrasion

Of all the various methods of eliminating or reducing acne scars, dermabrasion is the most widely used. According to dermatologists and plastic surgeons who perform dermabrasion, however, fewer dermabrasions are now being done than in years past. There are several reasons for this. First, many patients, anticipating miracles, are disappointed with the results. Second, collagen injections (discussed below), although not a permanent method of eliminating scars, have blunted the need for the more radical technique of dermabrasion. Finally, improved medications, particularly the development of the drug

Repairing the Damage: Scars

Accutane, have decreased the number of patients with scarring severe enough to warrant dermabrasion.

As the name implies, dermabrasion is a technique that removes the upper layers of the skin by a process of abrasion. The dermatologist uses equipment similar to a dental drill, a handle attached to an electrically powered motor. The rapidly spinning end of the handle is fitted with a steel wheel equipped with multiple small wires called a wire brush or a wheel impregnated with tiny diamond chips called a diamond fraise. The spinning brush or fraise scrapes away skin tissue to the desired depth.

If you choose to undergo dermabrasion, the procedure is performed in an operating room in the doctor's office or an outpatient facility. The procedure takes place while you are awake; the dermatologist uses ice packs and a spray-on anesthetic to numb and freeze the skin, which provides both the benefit of anesthesia and a firm surface that is more easily dermabraded. The areas to be treated are frozen and abraded in sections. Generally the entire face is abraded, but occasionally a localized area of scarring is treated by what is called "spot" dermabrasion.

The scars that are most likely to be improved by dermabrasion are those that are soft in consistency, with a scooped-out appearance. Actually, the scar is not being removed. What the dermatologist attempts to do is to abrade the surrounding normal tissue to the level of the scar, creating a more gradual slope at the margin, thus eliminating or modifying the appearance of holes and pits in the skin.

Postoperative care is very important. When the dermabrasion is completed, the skin is swollen, red, and raw, oozing serum. Some physicians apply specialized dressings that absorb the fluid, whereas others prefer to keep the skin exposed and clean, periodically removing the crusts that tend to form. Antibiotic salves are often applied to prevent infection. If all goes well, healing will be complete in two to three weeks, although the skin remains red and sensitive for several months. During this period you must

TREATING ACNE

avoid sun exposure so as not to develop ugly blotchy pigmentation of the abraded skin.

To fully appreciate what dermabrasion can do to eliminate acne scars, it's necessary to compare the depth of the abrasion with the depth of skin burns, which are rated as first-, second-, and third-degree injuries.

A *first-degree* burn is superficial; the injury is only to the epidermis. A sunburn that produces redness and peeling is a first-degree burn. Obviously a first-degree dermabrasion might eliminate some discolorations but would do nothing for acne scars. A *second-degree* burn extends into the upper portion of the dermis. Blistering occurs, but the injury is not deep enough to cause scarring. A *third-degree* burn, on the other hand, destroys so much of the dermis that scar tissue replaces the burned skin in the healing process.

The dermabrasion procedure seeks the second-degree level—it attempts to remove some dermis to level out scars but not to remove dermis to the depth of forming new scar tissue in the process. Unfortunately, many postacne scars, such as "ice pick" scars, extend deep into the dermis and therefore cannot be eliminated by dermabrasion. It is this limitation that causes some of the dissatisfaction with the procedure; deep scars may be improved, but they won't be eliminated. It is up to the skilled dermabrasion surgeon to assess the character and depth of your scars and candidly tell you the amount of improvement you can expect from the procedure.

Complications. There are a number of potential complications to dermabrasion, the most frequent of which is the loss of normal skin pigment once healing has taken place. If the dermabraded area, usually the whole face, is lighter than the rest of your skin, it will not be very obvious except under the chin and perhaps at the hairline. But it could be unsightly if the loss of pigment is spotty, with pale areas of skin mixed in with normally pigmented skin. This kind of

Repairing the Damage: Scars   71

pigment loss can usually be concealed with carefully applied makeup.

The opposite situation, too much pigmentation, can also occur. This complication can be caused by sun exposure during the healing phase, when the skin is pink and still sensitive. Often this type of excess pigment fades, like the pigmentation of a suntan, but sometimes it persists in a blotchy pattern that is difficult to conceal with makeup. If after a reasonable period of waiting the brown discoloration fails to fade, try treating it with the bleaching medication hydroquinone. This medication is sometimes used with a topical corticosteroid cream and Retin A to enhance its effectiveness. Unfortunately it is not always effective, even after months of use.

Another complication of dermabrasion is the forming of milia during healing. These white pimples are actually tiny cysts filled with an oily, seedlike plug. Milia can develop for no apparent reason, or as part of the acne condition, but when they appear during the healing process after dermabrasion there may be dozens or more of them. If they do not disappear spontaneously, a dermatologist can puncture them with a scalpel and squeeze out the contents.

The most feared complication of dermabrasion is, of course, scarring. Replacing old scars with new ones is discouraging at best. New scar formation can occur for two reasons: (1) if infection or some other inflammation complicates healing or (2) if the surgeon dermabrades too deeply and enters the third-degree zone. Scarring due to overdermabrading often occurs around the mouth or at the jawline. This type of scarring can be reduced or eliminated by applying corticosteroid cream or ointment at the site or by injecting it directly into the developing scar.

Occasionally individuals will develop a persistent flush after dermabrasion, due to a supersensitivity of the blood vessels of the face. This side effect usually subsides after a number of months. If it fails to disappear, it can usually be concealed with appropriate makeup.

TREATING ACNE

In summary, it is worth stressing that dermabrasion is still the most effective method of permanently modifying acne scars. It does, however, have its limitations. It is important that you understand all this, as well as the possible complications, since most of the dissatisfaction with the procedure arises from the patient's unrealistic expectations.

Excising Scars

It would be ideal if doctors could eliminate scars simply by cutting them out. Unfortunately, cutting into the skin incites the formation of more scar tissue. Some scars can be improved by removing them surgically, but many are made worse, with a larger or more obvious scar replacing a less prominent one. Elevated scars lend themselves to improvement through surgery, whereas flat or depressed ones do not.

A favorite method of dermatologists for removing small scars is to cut them out with a punch, an instrument that looks like a tiny cookie cutter. The circular cutting blade of the punch, measuring only a few millimeters in diameter, is pressed and rotated through the skin around the scar, thus removing a cone-shaped piece of skin and fat that encompasses the scar tissue.

There are several techniques of punch-excising scars. One consists of punching out small, ice pick–type scars and allowing the resulting hole to fill in with a blood clot and eventually a new scar. Generally the new scar is cosmetically a good tradeoff for the more obvious ice pick hole. A second method punches out a depressed scar, but, instead of removing it completely, simply elevates it to skin level, where it is taped or sutured in place. When healing is complete, you have a new scar, but as it is now flush with the skin surface, it is not so obvious. The third technique is more elaborate. It consists of punching out a scar and replacing it with a punched-out skin graft usually obtained

Repairing the Damage: Scars 73

from an area that is not readily visible, such as from the skin behind the ears. Such grafts take very well, but sometimes the skin doesn't match and occasionally the grafts cause scarring during healing or become discolored and unsightly.

Most excision of scars is done in conjunction with dermabrasion, sometimes at the same time or weeks before. Today, by and large, scar excision is a minor method of eliminating or reducing acne scars.

Chemical Peels

The application of caustic chemicals that irritate or chemically burn the skin and cause peeling is a cosmetic procedure that is used most frequently to treat aging and sun-damaged skin. These peels remove discolorations and superficial growths and blunt the appearance of minor wrinkles. Peels are less frequently performed to treat acne scarring because the majority of acne scars are deeper than the tissue removed by a peel, and are therefore more amenable to dermabrasion.

Some dermatologists use mild chemicals to perform light peels as a form of exfoliant therapy, preferring this method to freezing the skin with carbon dioxide (dry ice) or liquid nitrogen. Deeper peels that are designed to eliminate permanent marks and scars are more serious procedures and require sedation and a local anesthetic. The peeling agent, usually trichloroacetic acid or phenol, is then applied to the skin with cotton swabs. The chemical selected to induce the peel and its concentration determine the depth of the peel. Deeper peels obviously remove deeper wrinkles or scars. The depth can be increased by repeated applications of the peeling agent or by covering the skin with tape that is removed a day or two after the peel. The pain following a chemical peel can be severe, but it rarely lasts more than eight to twelve hours and is responsive to pain medication.

TREATING ACNE

Like dermabrasion, postoperative care depends on the philosophy of the doctor. Some surgeons apply antibiotic powder, encouraging a thick crust to form. Most believe that healing is enhanced by keeping the skin moist and so opt for soap and water cleansing and the application of antibiotic ointment. Immediately after the peel, the skin is red, swollen, and oozing, with considerable shedding of dead skin cells. From this stage to a healed but pink skin takes about two weeks.

The complications of a chemical peel are similar to the potential problems of dermabrasion. The moist, oozing skin is particularly susceptible to infection, which can lead to scarring. Thus, postoperative care to prevent infection is important. Loss of pigment in the peeled skin or the development of too much pigment weeks or months after the skin is healed is also common. Persistent redness of the skin and scarring, particularly around the mouth, occur less frequently.

It is worth restating that for modifying or eliminating the deep scars associated with acne, dermabrasion is a more predictable procedure than a chemical peel. Peels are used more as a form of exfoliant therapy and to remove the impermanent marks left by blemishes.

Filling Agents

The concept of modifying wrinkles and scars by filling them in with an injectable substance has been explored for years. In the last ten years, it has become particularly popular as a method of eliminating signs of aging and, to a lesser extent, scars.

Collagen. Collagen is the fibrous protein that makes up most of the connective tissue that constitutes the vast portion of our skin. Since scar tissue is also made up of collagen, the concept of adding more collagen to the scar area to improve its appearance seems like a reasonable approach.

Repairing the Damage: Scars

The material used by dermatologists and plastic surgeons to fill in scars is obtained from bovine (cow) collagen and marketed under the names Zyderm and Zyplast. Since some people are allergic to proteins that are not of human origin, you must be skin-tested before treatment. This is done by injecting a small amount of the collagen preparation into the skin on your forearm. A positive reaction—a firm red nodule at the injection site—may appear in a few days, or it may take three to four weeks. Approximately 3 percent of individuals have a positive reaction and are therefore disqualified for collagen treatment.

Once it has been demonstrated that you have no allergy to bovine collagen, treatment can begin. The collagen is injected through a fine needle into the line, furrow, or scar. In the case of acne, the scars that can be improved with collagen are the soft scars with gradually sloping borders, those that can be manually flattened by gently stretching the skin. Very firm scars with steep walls, such as ice pick scars, are not helped by this technique. Injecting the collagen into the skin level where it remains and provides maximum filling ensures the best results.

Although many acne scars lend themselves to correction with collagen, the improvement is not permanent. Over a period of months the collagen gradually disappears from the injection site. Within nine months to a year the scar again becomes apparent and a touch-up treatment is necessary to maintain the original improvement.

Another disappointing feature of collagen injections is the cost. Certainly dermabrasion is expensive, but it is a one-time outlay; collagen injections are an ongoing expense. Treating a few scars might require a syringe full of collagen, which costs several hundred dollars. Multiply this by the number of scars to be treated and re-treated, and it is easy to see that treatment and maintenance can run into the thousands of dollars. Yet despite the necessity for ongoing treatments and the expense involved, collagen

TREATING ACNE

injections are extremely popular and many thousands are administered every year.

Like any medication or treatment, there are possible side effects. Immediately after the injection there may be bruising, but these black and blue marks quickly go away; rarely does the skin break down due to the pressure of the volume of material injected. Allergic reactions to the collagen can occur even though your pretreatment skin test was negative. When this happens, itchy red bumps appear at the injection sites. Ultimately these often unattractive swellings persist for months despite treatment with corticosteroid medications. Some collagen recipients experience redness and swelling at the injection sites that appear to be triggered by sun exposure, exercise, or eating certain foods. These distressing problems may continue for several years, but they eventually disappear.

There have been recent reports that a number of collagen recipients had developed dermatomyositis, a rare skin and muscle disease, or polymyositis, a rare disease of the muscles. The FDA has an ongoing investigation of the possible connection between collagen treatments and these diseases, but so far they have insufficient evidence to link them. The manufacturer of collagen has always suggested that anyone with connective tissue disease, such as certain forms of arthritis, lupus erythematosus, and polymyositis, not be treated with collagen for fear of aggravating these illnesses.

Silicone. Silicone is a polymer, a compound made up of attached multiple molecules that contain the element silicon. Most of us are familiar with silicone because of its lubricating properties—it is used in medical products to lubricate syringes and coat the insides of blood tubes, in consumer products as a lubricant for door runners, and as an emollient in various cosmetics.

A special form of purified, sterile silicone has been used for some time by doctors as a filling agent. Since it has not been approved by the FDA, only a limited number of phy-

Repairing the Damage: Scars 77

sicians use silicone instead of collagen. The reasons for silicone's failure to gain FDA approval are complex, but they include patients' reactions to silicone preparations that may be related to impurities in the product or to errors in delivery technique rather than to the silicone itself.

There are some obvious advantages of silicone as a filling agent. Pure silicone does not initiate any allergic reactions. Furthermore, unlike collagen, it is permanent. Once injected into the skin, it remains indefinitely and, in fact, expands as new fibrous tissue grows around it. Doctors who use silicone for scars know that they must undercorrect—that is, not fill in the scar completely—since the silicone, plus the new tissue it attracts, can result in an unsightly bulge.

Silicone users state that side effects are minimal. But until large numbers of people are treated with a single uniform silicone product, it remains difficult to determine its risks.

Microlipoinjection. Liposuction has become a popular technique for removing the fat from thighs, buttocks, under the chin, and other areas of the body. It is a form of cosmetic "remodeling" accomplished by inserting a tube through an incision in the skin and sucking out the fat tissue with a vacuumlike apparatus. An offshoot technique of liposuction utilizes the fat removed to fill in depressions created by overvigorous fat removal. This has evolved into a technique called "microlipoinjection."

Under local anesthetic, fat is obtained from the thigh, buttock, abdomen, or elsewhere by aspirating it through a large needle inserted into the fat reservoir. The fat cells thus obtained can be used immediately or refrigerated for several weeks. A defect in the skin, such as an acne scar, can be corrected by injecting the fat into the scar, again through a large needle. Usually the scar is overcorrected—that is, filled in to the swelling point—since much of what is injected is fluid, which rapidly dissipates.

Since the fat used in microlipoinjection is your own tissue and not foreign material, allergic reactions do not occur. Two injection procedures are performed, withdrawing the fat and injecting it into the defect, so there is risk of infection if sterile procedures are not followed, but by and large it is a safe method. The major problem is that, like collagen injections, it is not permanent. Often after a year or so, the fat graft is lost or significantly reduced in two out of three individuals treated with this technique.

Fibrin. The newest filler to come along utilizes fibrin, a natural substance found in the blood. Fibrin is a critical material in normal blood clotting and wound healing. The technique involves injecting a mixture of gelatin (a protein substance obtained from pigs), a chemical called epsilon aminocaproic acid, and some of your own fibrin. A special type of cutting needle is used for the injection. It causes an injury at the scar site that stimulates the local cells to release chemicals that contribute to the formation of a clot made up of the injected gelatin and fibrin. The clot serves as a scaffold that attracts collagen-manufacturing cells into the area. Eventually the clot is replaced with collagen.

Since the gelatin is obtained from pigs and is thus a foreign protein, a skin test is necessary to make sure a patient does not suffer an allergic reaction. But in fact, allergy has not been a problem, and people who have become allergic to collagen through treatments are usually not allergic to the material used in fibrin treatments.

Side effects of fibrin injections are minimal. Some recipients experience temporary swelling and redness at the injection sites; others develop nodules that can persist for weeks. Hyperpigmentation—darkening of the skin—can occur that may or may not be permanent.

Perhaps the biggest selling point of the fibrin technique over collagen is its lasting quality. Whereas collagen lasts only for months to a year, fibrin correction is said to persist for up to five years. On the downside, fibrin injections improve the defect in only about 60 percent of those treated

Repairing the Damage: Scars

and few experience complete elimination of injected scars.

In summary, filling agents leave a lot to be desired. However, the risks involved in undergoing a series of injections are minimal, particularly when compared to some of the surgical methods described. It seems that the next few years will see an improvement in filling agents and the techniques available to deliver them and make them long lasting.

7

If It's Not Acne, What Is It?

You've probably heard the old saying: If it looks like a duck, walks like a duck, and quacks like a duck, then it must be a duck. Most of us have come to realize that this is not always the case. Doctors, in particular, are wary of the obvious. Every diagnosis summons up a mental list of other illnesses that might produce the same symptoms as the obvious cause of the disease. This process of sifting through the possibilities is called "considering the differential diagnosis."

Even a skin disease as familiar and commonplace as acne has a differential diagnosis. Most of the conditions that simulate acne have some obvious features that tell the careful observer that he or she is dealing with something other than acne. Thus it is useful for you to be familiar with some of these conditions.

ACNE ROSACEA

Sometimes simply called "rosacea," this condition is a malfunction of the small blood vessels in the part of the face where flushing occurs—the "T" zone that includes the cheeks, the mid-forehead, the nose, and chin. These blood vessels, which are particularly sensitive, enlarge when stimulated by heat and emotional factors. In people who suffer from acne rosacea, what starts as an increased flushing or blushing reaction from appropriate stimuli progresses to a persistent redness, a pattern of visible small veins in the red areas, and eventually to the presence of acne blemishes. Persistent, advanced rosacea causes a thickening of the skin, perhaps due to increased blood flow. This is most obvious on the nose, which increases in size and becomes coarse in appearance because of the formation of these irregular bumps and blemishes. This condition, rhinophyma, is familiar to most people as the "W. C. Fields nose," after the actor and comedian who was known for his bulbous nose.

The cause of rosacea is a mystery. It appears to be more a pattern of reaction in predisposed individuals than a disease with a specific cause. It occurs most often in fair-skinned individuals over thirty and in women more often than men.

The acne part of acne rosacea may not become apparent for years. When acne lesions finally do appear, they consist of red papules and pustules alone or they may accompany the red skin. Comedones are not present, which differentiates acne rosacea from a case of ordinary acne.

Any effective treatment of acne rosacea means the patient must avoid a number of aggravating factors. Dietary restrictions include the avoidance of hot liquids (coffee and tea should be drunk warm rather than steaming hot), spicy foods such as chili, and alcohol. (Rosacea and rhinophyma are aggravated but *not* caused by alcohol intake. Many individuals who suffer from rosacea and its cosmetic complications are teetotalers.) Exposure to the sun and extremes of temperature, either cold or hot, can also aggravate rosacea, as can emotional factors, both positive and negative. It's said that a cocktail party in a congested, over-

If It's Not Acne, What Is It?

heated room is a rosacea sufferer's nightmare—all of the aggravating factors are present that tend to dilate the blood vessels in the flushed area and increase the blood flow to the skin.

For reasons that are not clear, acne rosacea responds to antibiotics. Topical antibiotics like clindamycin and erythromycin are not as effective as oral tetracycline, which not only eliminates the acne lesions but also sometimes diminishes the redness. Other external treatments include corticosteroids, which must be used cautiously. They do decrease the redness initially, but prolonged use of the more potent corticosteroid creams can actually increase the development of the small dilated veins that are the hallmark of rosacea.

The newest medication used to treat rosacea is called metronidazole gel. When applied over a period of a few weeks, it decreases the formation of acne lesions and improves the red rash. Like tetracycline, the reasons for its effectiveness in acne rosacea are unknown.

The persistent, often disfiguring changes caused by long-standing uncontrolled acne rosacea can also be modified by surgery. Electrosurgery with a fine needle can eliminate the small veins, and other surgical methods, including laser surgery, have proved successful in remodeling a nose disfigured by rhinophyma.

It is not usually difficult to differentiate acne rosacea from true acne. The age of the afflicted is one clue. Although adult-onset acne is not uncommon, it is increasingly so after age thirty. The absence of comedones and the presence of fixed redness also speak in favor of acne rosacea. Occasionally the acne part of acne rosacea appears early and is more prominent than the redness, which may be perceived as merely "good coloring." Furthermore, it is possible for patients with protracted adult acne to develop acne rosacea in their thirties, which may lead to a mistaken diagnosis of a persistent adult acne condition.

PERIORAL DERMATITIS

Perioral dermatitis is a rash that occurs around the mouth. Often it resembles acne—small pimples and pustules erupt on red, inflamed skin. Sometimes it manifests itself as a red, dry, flaky rash.

Although new diseases are often variations of old ones, a description of perioral dermatitis was not found in the medical textbooks twenty-five years ago. It occurs predominantly in young women, and nobody knows where it comes from. At first it was believed that the persistent use of strong corticosteroid creams and ointments for other skin problems caused the rash, but studies show that most individuals with the problem did not use these medications before the eruption appeared. Similarly, cosmetics and fluoride toothpastes have not proven to be causal agents. To many dermatologists, perioral dermatitis appears to be a combination of acne and seborrheic dermatitis, a red, scaly rash that occurs on the scalp and face in areas with the greatest density of sebaceous glands.

Despite our admitted ignorance of its cause, perioral dermatitis, like acne, responds dramatically to antibiotics, particularly tetracycline. Not only do the acnelike blemishes disappear, but the redness and flaking clear up as well. Even with this impressive response to treatment, it is not unusual for the rash to recur sporadically over a period of years.

INFECTIONS

Several skin infections can mimic acne. The most common is folliculitis, an infection of the hair follicles. Men develop folliculitis more frequently than women, particularly in the beard area of the face.

The appearance of red pimples and pustules without the presence of comedones is suggestive of folliculitis. On close examination, it can be seen that each blemish devel-

If It's Not Acne, What Is It?

ops around a hair follicle. Unlike acne, the pimples of folliculitis are apt to be tender or painful.

Sometimes this infection is a complication of acne treatment. The sudden appearance of many small pus pimples may occur in acne patients who have been taking tetracycline or some other antibiotic for a long time; a strain of bacteria has developed in the follicles that is resistant to the antibiotic. These resistant bacteria thrive and multiply, and the infection appears. Treatment means switching to a different class of antibiotic, such as a form of penicillin or a sulfa drug.

Folliculitis that occurs independently of acne is often due to a staphylococcus infection. Treatment again is an antibiotic, such as a penicillin derivative, cephalosporin, or erythromycin. Shaving hygiene is an important part of treatment. Washing with an antibacterial soap or applying alcohol before and after shaving with a disposable razor can prevent spreading the infection with every shave.

Two viral infections are also occasionally mistaken for acne. Dozens of small warts, sometimes called "flat warts," can spread over the face in an acne pattern. It often takes a discerning eye to differentiate these skin-colored small bumps from comedones or acne papules. Unfortunately flat warts are difficult to eliminate. Dermatologists often prescribe Retin A because of its irritating properties. If effective, the warts become inflamed and then dry up and disappear. Should Retin A fail to work, cryosurgery (freezing) is usually an effective alternative.

Molluscum contagiosum is the other viral infection that can be mistaken for acne. As the name implies, this infection spreads easily on the skin surface, from one person to another. Each of the smooth pink papules of molluscum has a central depression, not always easy to see, that differentiates it from an acne papule or comedone. Molluscum papules have to be eliminated individually by a dermatologist, either by scraping them off with a sharp instrument called a skin curette or by destroying them by freezing or by using a caustic chemical.

HEAT RASH

Prickly heat, or miliaria, is characterized by a rash of small red pimples and sometimes pustules in areas of the skin where sweat glands are numerous, such as the face and torso. It is usually distinguishable from acne because its abrupt appearance is associated with sweating or exposure to heat and humidity. Actually, heat rash and acne have a similar origin. Heat rash is due to blockage of the sweat ducts; acne results from blockage of the follicular ducts. Sometimes heat rash develops in acne patients, creating the impression that the acne is suddenly flaring. Heat rash is usually short-lived if the individual is placed in a cool, low-humidity environment.

CONTACT ALLERGY

Allergic reactions that appear on the face are rarely confused with acne. Contact allergy is an itchy rash made up of papules and sometimes blisters, although no comedones or pustules are present. The areas of skin involved correspond to where the allergic substance has touched the skin, which may differ from the normal pattern of an acne eruption.

The one situation in which confusion may arise occurs when an acne medication, such as benzoyl peroxide, causes an allergic reaction. Often the allergic rash, superimposed on the acne, is interpreted as a sudden worsening of the acne itself. If not recognized for what it is, continued use of the medication-allergen only makes things worse. On the other hand, discontinuation of the acne treatments will soon clarify the situation.

Finally, there are times when the saying about the duck does apply: What looks and acts like acne *is* acne. For example, when someone who has consistently clear skin sud-

If It's Not Acne, What Is It?

denly erupts with pimples and pustules, he or she should consider the possibility that there may be an inciting cause for the outbreak. If immediately recognized and treated, the condition might clear up without prolonged therapy. In such a case, ask yourself the following questions:

- Are you using any new cosmetics, such as a moisturizer or oily foundation, that could have triggered the acne outbreak?

- Has there been any change in your life that might cause an alteration of the androgen/estrogen balance, such as discontinuing birth control pills or even childbirth itself? Have there been any other physical changes that suggest increased androgen activity, such as an irregular menstrual cycle or abnormal hair growth?

- Are there any occupational or environmental changes that would favor the development of certain types of acne, such as athletic friction acne, acne cause by oil particles in the atmosphere, or chloracne?

- Are you taking any medications that can cause acne, such as androgen or corticosteroid hormones, iodine or other halogens, lithium, or antiepileptic medications?

Discovering and eliminating any of these causal factors might very well solve an acne problem in people who are not usually acne-prone.

8

Finding Professional Help

Acne is not always a minor problem with simple, surefire methods of treatment. If you have a mild case of acne, you may very well be satisfied with what you have learned here about its cause and treatment and elect to handle the problem yourself. If so, then this book has accomplished one of its major purposes. If you have more severe acne, or an acne condition that has failed to respond to an adequate program of self-treatment, or if you don't choose to deal with your skin condition yourself, you may opt for professional help.

There are several reasons for turning to a dermatologist for advice about the treatment of acne.

WHY SEE A SPECIALIST?

If experience is the best teacher, dermatologists have seen hundreds, if not thousands, of patients with acne and are singularly well equipped to evaluate this problem. A dermatologist can identify the type of acne, assess its severity, select the appropriate treatment, and venture an informed opinion about your response to treatment and the overall outlook.

If you have a mild case of acne and have not been successful with over-the-counter medications, a visit to the dermatologist is indicated. After providing information and outlining a treatment plan, the doctor may encourage you to go it alone and return only if treatment is not successful or if the condition worsens.

If you have more severe acne or need the support and attention of sustained care, follow-up visits are appropriate. When internal medications are prescribed, follow-up visits are mandatory so that the doctor can evaluate the medication's effectiveness and any side effects and adjust the dosage when necessary. If left to their own devices, many patients cling to medications that may no longer be required or have lost their efficacy. This is one reason why doctors are reluctant to keep refilling prescriptions without a face-to-face evaluation of the status of your acne.

When to Seek Professional Help

There is considerable overlap between the why and the when to seek help. With a case of mild acne, it is appropriate to find help if self-treatment is not doing all that it should, although it is possible to be premature in making this decision. Many do-it-yourselfers are impatient when valid over-the-counter medications fail to resolve their acne in a few days or in a week or two. They fail to realize that medications that alter the causes of acne take weeks and sometimes months to produce sustained improvement.

If you have more severe acne, help becomes essential as soon as it is obvious that self-treatment is not controlling the acne and something stronger, a prescription medication, is required. In the case of recognizable cystic acne, it

Finding Professional Help

is recommended that the do-it-yourself approach be by-passed in favor of immediate professional attention. All too often cystic acne sufferers go to a dermatologist after scarring has already occurred. Treatment at that stage will prevent further scarring but will not reverse much of the damage that has already been done.

In summary, professional care is indicated when self-treatment is not effective, when previously controlled self-treated acne flares or becomes unresponsive to home treatment, and when acne is so severe at the outset that it demands more drastic treatment than over-the-counter medications can provide.

How to Choose a Doctor

People differ in their methods of choosing a physician. At one extreme is the "supermarket" approach, in which location, convenience, and cost are the determining factors. At the other extreme, which might be called "the best is none too good" approach, careful selection is followed by a trial appointment-interview in which the patient assesses the doctor's qualities. Most people take a middle approach. They are looking for a competent doctor with whom they will feel comfortable. They ask their friends with similar problems and values, or call on their family physician for a referral.

If these sources are not available, you can call your local hospital, your county or state medical society, the American Medical Association, or, in the case of dermatology, the American Academy of Dermatology, 1567 Maple Avenue, P.O. Box 3166, Evanston, IL 60204-3166, (312) 869-3954.

Once you select a physician, it is important to keep in mind that a first visit does not establish an eternal, permanent relationship. You always have the option of "divorcing" your doctor and finding another, although many people are reluctant to do so. (Doctors, on the other hand,

TREATING ACNE

find it difficult to get rid of patients and not be charged with abandonment.) It might seem as if most acne treatment is standard, but there are extreme differences in treatment philosophy among dermatologists. For example, some specialists start with the mildest form of therapy, working up to stronger medications if the less potent versions fail to do the job. Others prefer strong treatment at the outset, no matter what the severity of the acne, and work down to milder medications once the acne is under control.

Another major difference in treatment practices concerns the use of physical forms of therapy. There are dermatologists who regularly perform acne surgery or freeze or peel the skin with acid. Others rarely, if ever, use these methods. All dermatologists have seen patients who left one of their colleagues because there was too much or not enough of these physical treatments. Like the doctors themselves, patients differ in their appraisal of these methods, and many use it as a factor in selecting or leaving a physician.

Obviously communication is the most important aspect of a satisfactory patient-doctor relationship. The doctor should encourage you to ask questions, express your concerns, and contribute to decisions about your therapy. You in turn must be honest with your doctor about your compliance with his or her instructions. Nothing is more wasteful and disheartening than repeated changes in treatment because of an apparent lack of improvement, when in fact the patient is not really following the treatment plan. In short, if both you and your physician are honest and open with each other, the therapy stands a good chance of success.

Glossary

Acne: a skin disease that affects the hair follicles and sebaceous glands on the face, chest, and back and that is characterized by a variety of different blemishes.

Acnegenic: causing acne to develop.

Androgen: male hormone produced by the adrenal glands, testes, and ovaries.

Astringent: an alcohol lotion that dries the skin and produces a tight sensation.

Collagen: a natural fibrous protein found in the skin and used by injection to repair scars.

Comedogenic: causing the formation of comedones.

Comedone: a blackhead or whitehead; an obstructing plug inside the pilosebaceous duct.

Cryotherapy: freezing the skin to reduce inflammation or to promote peeling.

Cyst: a sacklike structure usually filled with fluid or semisolid material, such as a sebaceous cyst.

Cyst (acne): large acne blemishes deep within the skin.

Dermabrasion: a surgical method to reduce acne scars by abrading away part of the skin.

TREATING ACNE

Estrogen: female hormone produced by the ovaries.

Exfoliant: a substance that makes the skin peel.

Exfoliate: to peel off (the skin).

Folliculitis: inflammation or infection of hair follicles.

Hormone: a chemical produced by the endocrine glands that is carried by the blood to various parts of the body, where it regulates metabolic and other functions.

Hyperpigmentation: a darkening of the skin usually due to an increase in melanin.

Keloid: an unusually thick and often oddly shaped scar.

Lipid: referring to fatty substances.

Melanin: the pigment that gives skin its color; its presence increases with exposure to the sun.

Milia: tiny whitish pimples that are actually small cysts.

Miliaria: heat rash.

Papule: a solid swelling on the skin surface; a pimple.

Pustule: a small abscess, a pimple filled with pus.

Sebaceous gland: the gland that is attached to the hair follicle that produces sebum.

Sebum: an oily substance that lubricates and protects the skin surface.

Index

A

Abrasive cleansers, 29, 31, 65
Accutane, 49–54, 56–58, 68–69
Acne
  adult, 12
  athletic, 13, 14, 87
  causes of, 13–15, 17–25
  climate and, 22–23
  cosmetics and, 12, 38, 59–66
  cystic, 9, 10, 21, 31, 34, 42, 44,
    50, 53–58, 67, 71, 90–91
  definition of, 5
  diet and, 12, 23–24, 34, 82
  differential diagnosis, 81–87
  emergencies, 35–36
  genetic factors, 18
  infantile, 11–12
  medications causing, 14–15,
    87
  myths and truths of, 21–25
  occupational, 13–14, 87
  pathogenesis of, 17
  pregnancy and, 45, 51, 57
  professional help for, 89–92
  scars and. See Scars
  steroid, 20
  sun, 22

  symptoms of, 6–11
  treatment of. See Treatments
Acne conglobata, 12–13
Acne excoriée, 24–25
Acne fulminans, 13
Acne rosacea, 81–83
Acne surgery, 54–56, 92
Adrenal glands, 19, 48, 49
Adult acne, 12
Alcohol, 82
Aluminum salts, 29
American Academy of
  Dermatology, 91
American Medical Association,
  91
Anabolic steroids, 14
Androgens, 19–20, 47, 87
Antiandrogens, 48–50
Antibiotics, 13, 34, 54, 63, 74
  cephalosporin, 85
  clindamycin, 42, 52, 83
  doxycycline, 45, 46, 52
  erythromycin, 42, 43, 45–46,
    52, 57, 83, 85
  meclocycline, 42, 43, 52
  minocycline, 45, 46, 52
  Nystatin, 44
  oral, 43–47, 52, 58, 83

Index

Antibiotics *(cont'd)*
  penicillin, 14, 46, 85
  tetracycline, 42, 44–47, 52, 83–85
  topical, 41–44, 52, 57, 58, 66, 83
Arthritis, 76
Astringents, 29–31, 37, 63, 66
Athletic acne, 13, 14, 87

B

Bacteria, 21, 22, 28, 31, 32, 42–46, 52, 85
Beauty salons, 37–38
Benzoyl peroxide, 28, 32–33, 36, 41, 43, 57, 58, 63, 65, 66, 86
Birth control pills, 14, 45, 47–48, 52, 87
Blackheads, 6–8, 11, 20, 22, 34, 35, 37, 40, 55
Bleaching creams, 10
Blushes, 64
Bromine, 13–15, 23–24
Butyl stearate, 62

C

Cancer, 22–23, 36, 54
Candida albicans fungus, 44
Cephalosporin, 85
Chemical peels, 67, 73–74, 92
Chicken pox, 5
Chili, 82
Chloracne, 14, 87
Chlorine, 13–14
Chocolate, 23
Cleaning skin, 22, 27–31, 65, 85
Climate, 22–23
Clindamycin, 42, 52, 83

Closed comedones, 6–8, 11, 20, 35, 37, 40, 55–56
Cocoa butter, 61, 62
Coconut oil, 61, 62
Coffee, 82
Collagen injections, 67, 68, 74–76
Comedogenic substances, 60–62
Comedone extractor, 35, 55
Comedones, 6–8, 11, 20, 21, 29, 31, 34, 40, 41, 55–56, 60–63, 67, 82–84
Contact allergy, 86
Corticosteroids, 13, 14, 20, 49–50, 53, 54, 56, 58, 71, 76, 83, 84, 87
Cosmetics, 12, 37–38, 59–66, 84, 87
Cryoroller, 53
Cryotherapy, 53–54, 85, 92
Cyproterone, 48
Cystic acne, 9, 10, 21, 31, 34, 42, 44, 50, 53–58, 67, 71, 90–91

D

D&C red dyes, 62, 64
Decyl oleate, 62
Deep cleansers, 38
Dermabrasion, 67–74
Dermatitis, 30, 84
Dermatologists, 89–92
Dermatomyositis, 76
Diet, 12, 23–24, 34, 82
Doxycycline, 45, 46, 52
Dry ice, 31–32, 53, 73
Ducts, 5–7

E

Eczema, 30
Electrical equipment, 14

Index

Electrosurgery, 83
Emergencies, 35–36
Emotional factors, 24–25, 82
Endocrine glands, 19
Environment, 12–14, 87
Epidermis, 20
Epsilon aminocaproic acid, 78
Erythromycin, 42, 43, 45–46, 52, 57, 83, 85
Estrogens, 14, 19, 20, 47–48, 52, 57, 87
Ethinyl estradiol, 47
Excising scars, 67, 72–73
Exfoliants, 31–32, 35, 40, 57, 58
Eye makeup, 64

F

Facials, 37–38
Fatty acids, 21
Fibrin injections, 78–79
Filling agents, 74–79
Flat warts, 85
Fluorine, 23–24
Follicles, 5, 20–23, 29, 31, 32, 35, 42, 46, 55, 56, 60, 84–85
Folliculitis, 84–85
Food and Drug Administration (FDA), 38, 40, 59, 76, 77
Foods, 23–24, 82
Foundations, 63–65, 87
French fried potatoes, 23
Fruit pits, 29

G

Gelatin, 78
Genetic factors, 18
Glyceryl stearate, 62

H

Halogen chemicals, 13–15, 23–24, 87
Heat rash, 86
Hives, 14, 46
Hormones, 11, 12, 14, 19–20, 47–50, 52–54, 57, 58, 87
Humidity, 23
Hydroquinone, 71
Hyperpigmentation, 10, 78

I

"Ice pick" scars, 10, 56, 70, 72, 75
Infantile acne, 11–12
Infections, 84–85
Insecticides, 14
Iodine, 15, 23–24, 87
Isoniazid, 15
Isopropyl isostearate, 62
Isopropyl myristate, 62, 63
Isopropyl palmitate, 62
Isotretinoin, 13, 49–53

K

Keloids, 10, 13, 54

L

Lanolin, 61, 62
Laser surgery, 83
Lipid-free cleansers, 30
Liposuction, 77
Lipstick, 64
Liquid nitrogen, 31–32, 53, 73
Lithium, 15, 87
Lupus erythematosus, 76

M

Macules, 9
Makeup sticks, 65
Masks, 37–38
Meclocycline, 42, 43, 52
Medicated soaps, 28, 29, 57, 58
Medication acne, 14–15, 87
Medications. *See* Antibiotics; Treatments
Melanin, 10
Metronidazole gel, 83
Microlipoinjections, 77–78
Milia, 55, 56, 71
Miliaria, 86
Mineral oil, 61, 63
Minocycline, 45, 46, 52
Moisturizers, 62–63, 87
Molluscum contagiosum, 85
Myristyl myristate, 62

N

Nonsoap cleansers, 30
Nystatin, 44

O

Occupational acne, 13–14, 87
Oily skin, 18–19
Olive oil, 61
Open comedones, 6–8, 11, 20, 22, 34, 35, 37, 40, 55
Oral antibiotics, 43–47, 52, 58, 83
Ovaries, 19, 48, 49
Overtreatment, 27

P

Papules, 7–9, 11, 21, 29, 31, 40–42, 44, 50, 54, 56, 60, 67, 82, 84–87
Peanut oil, 61
Peels, chemical, 67, 73–74, 92
Penicillin, 14, 46, 85
Perioral dermatitis, 84
Petrolatum, 62
Phenol, 73
Phenytoin, 15
Phlebitis, 47, 48
Physical therapy, 53–58, 92
Pilosebaceous ducts, 5, 6
Pimples. *See* Papules
Pizza, 23
Plastic, 14, 29
Pledgettes, 66
Polyethylene plastic, 29
Polymyositis, 76
Powders, 63–64
Pregnancy, 45, 51, 57
Prescribed treatments, 39–58
Prickly heat, 86
Primers, 65
Progesterone, 14
Propylene glycol monostearate, 62
Psoriasis, 37
Punch-excising scars, 72–73
Pus, 9, 12–13
Pustules, 9, 11, 21, 31, 34, 37, 40, 41, 44, 46, 53–57, 60, 67, 82, 84–87

R

"Rabbit ear" test, 60–61
Resorcinol, 31, 66
Retin A (retinoic acid), 40–41, 43, 52, 56–58, 63, 66, 71, 85

Index

Rhinophyma, 82, 83
Rosacea, 81–83

S

Saffron oil, 61
Salicylic acid, 31, 36, 65, 66
Scars, 9, 10, 13, 34, 35, 54–56, 91
   chemical peels, 67, 73–74, 92
   collagen injections, 67, 68, 74–76
   dermabrasion, 67–74
   excising, 67, 72, 73
   fibrin injections, 78–79
   microlipoinjections, 77–78
   silicone injections, 76–77
Sebaceous glands, 5, 7, 11, 14, 19, 20, 22, 32, 47, 52, 53, 57, 84
Seborrheic dermatitis, 84
Sebum, 5, 6, 9, 11, 19–21, 23, 28, 31, 47, 50, 54, 57
Self-surgery, 34–35
Self-treatments, 27–38
Shaving, 85
Side effects of treatments, 44–52, 70–71, 76–78
Silicone injections, 76–77
Sinus tracts, 13
Skin cancers, 22–23, 36, 54
Skin curette, 85
Skin hygiene, 22, 27–31, 65, 85
"Slush," 53
Soaps, 28–31, 57, 58, 65, 85
Sodium lauryl sulfate, 62
Spironolactone, 48, 53
Spot dermabrasion, 69
Staphylococcus infections, 85
Stearic acid, 62
Steroid acne, 20
Stress, 12, 24–25
Sulfa drugs, 46, 85
Sulfur, 31, 36, 66

Sun acne, 22
Sunflower oil, 61
Sunlamps, 36–37
Sunlight, 36, 45, 46, 82
Sunscreens, 41, 45, 59
Surgery, 54–56, 92

T

Tanning parlors, 37
Tea, 82
Testes, 19
Testosterone, 14
Tetracycline, 42, 44–47, 52, 83–85
Therapeutic cosmetics, 38
Thyroid gland, 19, 54
Thyroxin, 19
Toothpastes, 84
Topical antibiotics, 41–44, 52, 57, 58, 66, 83
Treatments, 65–66, 83, 91
   during pregnancy, 57
   prescribed, 39–58
   of scars. See Scar
   self-help, 27–38
   side effects of, 44–52, 70–71, 76–78
   See also Antibiotics
Tretinoin, 40–41, 43, 52, 56–58, 63, 66, 71, 85
Trichloroacetic acid, 73
Trimethoprim sulfamethoxazole, 45
"T" zone, 82

V

Vaginal yeast infections, 44–45
Vitamin A, 33–34, 40, 50

Vitamin supplements, 33–34
Vleminckx Solution, 31

W

Warts, 85
Washing skin, 22, 27–31, 65, 85
Weed killers, 14
White blood cells, 9, 21
Whiteheads, 6–8, 11, 20, 35, 37, 40, 55–56
Wire insulation, 14

X

X-ray therapy, 54

Y

Yogurt, 45

Z

Zinc, 34
Zyderm, 75
Zyplast, 75